Milady's
Nail Structure
&
Product Chemistry

Delmar Publishers' Online Services

To access Delmar on the World Wide Web, point your browser to: **http://www.delmar.com/delmar.html**
To access through Gopher: **gopher://gopher.delmar.com**

(Delmar Online is part of "thomson.com", an Internet site with information on more than 30 publishers
of the International Thomson Publishing organization.)
For information on our products and services:
email: info@delmar.com or   call **800-347-7707**

Milady's
Nail Structure
&
Product Chemistry

by
Douglas Schoon, M.S.

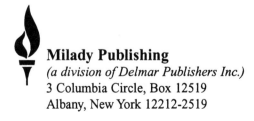

Milady Publishing
(a division of Delmar Publishers Inc.)
3 Columbia Circle, Box 12519
Albany, New York 12212-2519

NOTICE TO THE READER

Cover Design: Brian Yacur

Milady Staff
Publisher: Catherine Frangie
Acquisitions Editor: Joseph Miranda
Project Editor: Annette Downs Danaher
Production Manager: Brian Yacur

COPYRIGHT © 1996
Milady Publishing
(a division of Delmar Publishers)
an International Thomson Publishing company I(T)P

Printed in the United States of America
Printed and distributed simultaneously in Canada

For more information, contact:
Milady Publishing
3 Columbia Circle , Box 12519
Albany, New York 12212-2519

2 3 4 5 6 7 8 9 10 XXX 01 00 99 98

Library of Congress Cataloging-in-Publication Data

Schoon, Douglas D.
    Milady's nail structure and product chemistry/ Douglas Schoon
        p.   cm.   Includes Index.
    ISBN: 1-56253-239-1
    1. Manicuring. 2. Nails (Anatomy) – Care and hygiene.
    3. Fingernails. I. Milady Publishing Company. II. Title.
TT958.3.S36 1995   95-102229
646.7'27–dc20   CIP

A Dedication

For My Mother and Father

Thanks for my first chemistry set and everything else since.

Contents

Helpful Hints to Students

Learning any subject can be made easier. In many ways, going to school is like a job. The job of learning is up to each student, but there are ways to make the job easier and more enjoyable. The following advice will help you get the most from reading this book.

Although the book is designed to make it easier to learn, textbooks are not novels. You cannot expect to quickly read or skim each chapter and know everything. You must do some studying. These tips will help you learn.

1. Look for words in **boldface.**

While reading the chapters you will notice that some words are unfamiliar, Usually, these words will be **boldfaced.** Pay special attention to any word in **boldface and make sure you understand its meaning.**

2. Use the chapter summaries ("Fast Tracks") as a guide.

At the end of each chapter you will find a Fast Track, or chapter summary. These summaries review the most important idea from the chapter. Be sure to read the summaries several times. If you don't understand a topic, go back and reread that part of the chapter.

3. Don't just skip over what you don't understand.

There is no shame in asking your teacher to explain something you find difficult to understand. That's a teacher's job. Most teachers will be thrilled and impressed if you show a real interest in learning. Your future employers will see this desire to learn, as well. Nobody wants to hire people who think they know it all or have closed minds. Learn for the rest of your life! What you know can help your future, even save your life.

About the Author

Douglas Schoon obtained his master's degree in chemistry from the University of California–Irvine. He has more than 20 years of experience as a chemical researcher, lecturer, and educator. He is the president and founder of the Chemical Awareness Training Service, base in Newport Beach, California. Mr. Schoon has authored dozens of articles and lectured nationwide on the important topic of salon chemical safety.

As a research consultant for leading manufacturers, Mr. Schoon has developed many successful professional products for the beauty industry. He also serves as an expert witness in legal cases helping attorneys, judges, and juries to understand the chemical complexities of professional and retail beauty industry products.

Mr. Schoon is a member of the Nail Manufacturer's Council's Safety and Standards Committee (a division of the American Beauty Association), which is concerned with disinfection and sanitation safety and methods, as well as chemical safety.

Acknowledgments

I would like to thank Paul Rollins for the brilliant photographic work and drawings you see in this book. I would also like to thank Creative Nail Design Systems, Inc. for allowing me to use these photos and laboratory data. A special thanks to Corrine Dillard, who has probably read everything I have written in the last seven years, before it was corrected, and made sure it was right. Finally, I would like to thank Cathy Frangie, a great lady and the chief editor of Milady Publishing, for allowing me the chance to bring this much-needed information to nail technicians everywhere.

I am also grateful to the following reviewers who provided very useful suggestions and comments:

Judy Landis-Storm, Just My Imagination, Laguna Beach, CA

Jill Busler, Creative Nail Design Systems, Inc., Vista, CA

Diana Crosthwait, Salon Partners, Fort Worth, TX

Herman Paez, Lovetouch Salon, Denton, TX

Paula Gilmore, Tips Salon and Image Center, Redwood City, CA

Stella Niffenegger, Cincinnatti, OH

Betty Romesberg, Cuyahoga Falls, OH

Madeline Udod, Farmingville, NY

Barrie Allen, North Brentwood, NY

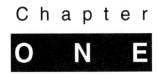

Fingernail Anatomy

What is the job of professional nail technicians? Is it to give clients beautiful, long-lasting, and durable artificial nail enhancements? No, the duty of every professional nail technician is to protect and nurture the fingernail. The health of the natural nail plate, bed, and surrounding tissue is your responsibility. You may find that your clients don't care about their natural nails. This is because they pay YOU to care. If nail health comes FIRST, then nail beauty will follow.

It can be tempting to ignore the health of the fingernail, but always remember, "Artificial Fingernails: *Enhancements* – Not Replacements!" A beautiful set of artificial nail enhancements is no replacement for diseased or lost fingernails. It is easy to keep your client's fingernails healthy, but it won't happen by accident. Knowledge is the key. The chapters on fingernail anatomy and health are presented first because they are the most important. Learn all you can about the fingernail and its many parts and you'll be the nail technician that everyone admires and respects. You'll have fewer problems and happier clients. You will be a true professional!

The Fingernail

Ask someone to show you one of their "fingernails." Usually they will point to the nail plate, the hard structure growing from the tip of the finger. Actually, the nail plate is only one of many parts of the fingernail. Some believe this is the most important part of the fingernail, but it isn't. The fingernail can be divided into seven major sections. Together these form what is called the **nail unit.** Figures 1.1 and 1.2 show drawings of the complete nail unit. Damage or disease to any part of the nail unit can spell trouble. Each is vital to maintaining a healthy fingernail.

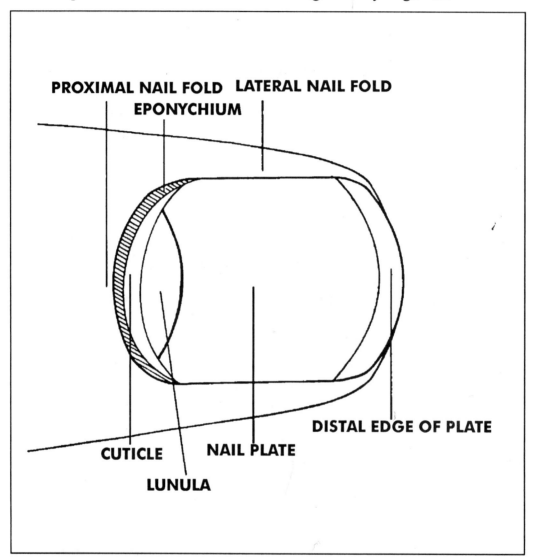

Fig. 1.1
Anatomy of the nail unit. *(Courtesy Paul Rollins.)*

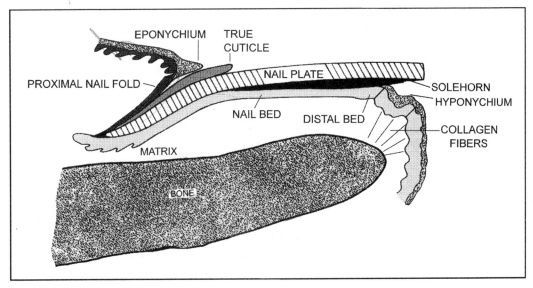

EPONYCHIUM   TRUE
             CUTICLE

PROXIMAL NAIL FOLD

NAIL PLATE

SOLEHORN
HYPONYCHIUM

NAIL BED   DISTAL BED

COLLAGEN
FIBERS

MATRIX

BONE

Fig. 1.2
Cross section of the nail unit. *(Courtesy Paul Rollins.)*

Parts of The Nail Unit

Nail Folds

The skin does not end at the nail plate. Instead it folds underneath and covers the emerging nail plate. This skin fold protects the new, emerging nail plate. This fold is part of the nail unit. It is called the **proximal nail fold.** Proximal means "nearest attached end." The skin on either side of the nail plate is an extension of the proximal nail fold, called the **lateral nail fold.** In this case, lateral means "to the side." Normally, the proximal nail fold has the appearance of smooth, healthy skin. It can be injured by cuts, nicks and bruises, or irritating chemicals. Once the proximal nail fold is damaged, bacteria, fungi, or viruses can attack and cause infection. The proximal nail fold forms a seal or barrier that protects the area where the nail plate is made.

Matrix

Directly below the proximal nail fold is a small area of living tissue called the **matrix.** *The matrix is the most important part of the nail unit.* The matrix produces cells that form the nail plate. These cells are much like those found in a shaft of hair.

The size and shape of the matrix determine the thickness and width of the nail plate. The wider the matrix area, the wider the nail plate. Therefore, the matrix of the thumb must be wider than the matrix area of the little finger. Also, longer matrices make thicker nail plates. A person who has naturally thin nail plates must have a very short matrix area. If the matrix becomes damaged in any way, the effects will be seen in the nail plate.

Cuticle and Eponychium

The cuticle is a part of the proximal nail fold. Specifically, it is the skin that touches the nail plate. There is more to the cuticle than what is visible. As you have learned, the skin curls underneath to form the proximal nail fold (see Figure 1.1). The skin underneath the fold is different than the visible top surface. The underside of the proximal nail fold constantly sheds a layer of colorless skin. This shed skin attaches to the topside of the emerging nail plate. It then "rides" on the nail plate and seems to grow from under the fold. This is the **true cuticle.** The visible skin fold that appears to end at the base of the nail plate is the **eponychium.** Sometimes, this tissue is incorrectly called the cuticle. During a manicure, the eponychium is gently pushed back to expose the true cuticle which should be carefully removed. You will see later that improperly performing this part of the manicure causes many problems for clients. It can lead to service breakdown of artificial nails and may seriously damage the nail unit.

Nail Plate

The nail plate is mostly **keratin,** the same chemical substance that forms hair. Keratin is a protein made from amino acids. These special proteins form a strong, flexible material which we call the nail plate. You will learn in Chapter 2 that nail plate formation is very similar to skin and hair growth. The nail plate is made of many layers of dead, flattened cells. These plate-like cells are cemented to each other with a sticky substance. When many layers stick to each other they form a structure that resembles a mortar and brick wall. The nail plate is also called the **natural nail.**

After a keratin cells grows in the matrix it is pushed outward and slightly upward by newer cells. The new growth emerges from under the proximal nail fold at the eponychium (see Figure 1.2). As new cells leave the matrix, they push the older cells toward the fingertips. Eventually, each keratin cell will reach the end of the finger. The part of the nail plate that grows beyond the fingertip is called the **free edge** or the **distal nail plate.** Distal means "farthest from the attached end." It is important to remember the difference between distal and proximal. Proximal means "nearest attached end". Therefore, distal is the opposite of proximal. These words may seem strange at first, but they are important to understand.

The hard keratin plate protects the nail bed and fingertip. Thicker nail plates provide greater protection. Obviously, if the nail plate is thinned too much, it cannot properly protect the delicate tissue underneath. This is often seen in nails that are overmanicured or filed. *Overfiling the natural nail is a leading cause of nail plate thinning and destruction.*

When keratin cells leave the matrix they are plump and whitish in appearance. Before emerging from under the eponychium the cells flatten, become transparent, and lose their color. This explains why nail plates are normally colorless, except for the white half-moon at the cuticle.

Lunula

The **lunula** (half-moon) is the whitish, opaque area at the base (proximal end) of the nail plate. The plump, white keratin cells flatten like pancakes. When they flatten, most of the material inside the cell is lost. This is why the cells become transparent. The lunula is formed by cells that have not yet completely flattened or lost their inner material. Not all fingers have a lunula. On fingers with a lunula, the front end of the matrix is directly below the whitish area. The lunula outlines the front part of the matrix. The lunula is usually seen on the thumb and index finger. Interestingly, you can tell if a person is right- or left-handed by which thumb has the largest lunula. The thumb with the largest lunula is on the dominant hand.

The lunula also determines the shape of the nail plate. Look at the shape of your lunula and compare it to the natural shape of the nail plate's free edge. They are an identical match. Both the lunula and free edge are crescent shaped. As mentioned above, it is also the shape of the distal (front end) part of the matrix. Animals with different-shaped lunulas have nails (or claws) which also match in shape. Figure 1.3 shows the claw and lunula shapes of six different types of primates.[1] Notice that the shape of the lunula closely matches the free edge.

---

[1]Drawing from LeGros, CWB, *The Problems of the Claw in Primates.* Proc. Zool Sovc. 1:1, 1936.

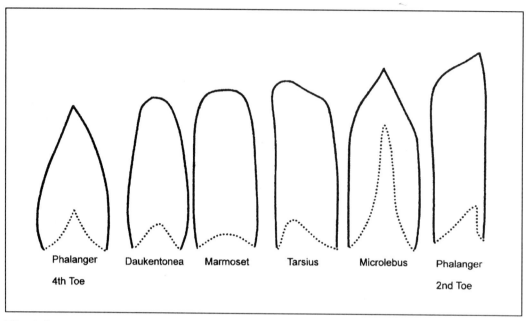

Fig. 1.3
Claw and lunula shape for six different primates. *(Courtesy Paul Rollins.)*

Nail Bed

The **nail bed** lies directly under the nail plate. It starts at the matrix and ends just before the free edge. Like skin, the nail bed is made of two types of tissue, **dermis** and **epidermis.** The dermis is the lower or basement layer of tissue (found just below the epidermis). The epidermis is the upper layer and is closest to the nail plate. These two skin layers have unique shapes. The dermis has many grooves or channels running from the lunula to just before the free edge. The epidermis has ridges or rails running the same direction. These ridges fit neatly into the channels found in the dermis as shown in Figure 1.4.

The dermis is attached to the bone underneath. Therefore, the dermis is locked into place and does not move. The epidermis is very different. It is firmly attached to the underside of the nail plate. So, the epidermis moves with the nail plate as it grows. This happens because the ridges of the epidermis are free to slide in the channels of the dermis.

As the nail plate grows, the channels act like many sets of train tracks, guiding the ridges of the epidermis. Besides keeping the nail plate "on track," the grooves also hold the ridges in place. This prevents the nail plate from lifting off the nail bed. The

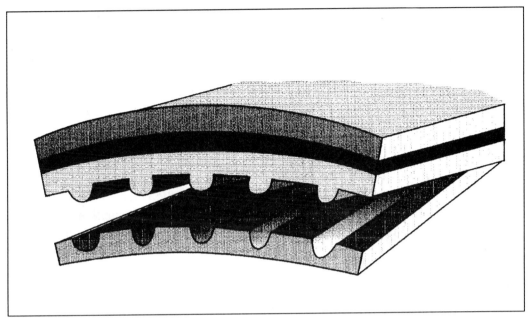

Fig. 1.4
This drawing shows how the rails on the bottom side of the epidermis fit into the grooves in the top surface of the nail bed. This arrangement allows the nail plate to glide across the surface of the nail bed as it grows. *(Courtesy Paul Rollins.)*

nail bed does not add keratin cells to the nail plate. All nail growth occurs in the matrix under the proximal nail fold and lunula.

Solehorn

The epidermis remains attached to the underside of the nail plate until it grows past the fingertip. This epidermis can be seen by closely examining the underside of the free edge. This is called the **solehorn** or **solehorn cuticle.** The solehorn usually sloughs away on its own or may be removed during a manicure.

Blood and Nerve Supply

A rich supply of nutrients is delivered to the nail unit by the blood. **Arteries** carry blood from the heart to other parts of the body. Two arteries supply each nail unit. A single artery runs along each side of the finger passing through the lateral nail fold. After leaving the nail fold, they run deep into the dermis (basement tissue) of the nail bed. Many small branches carry blood from the arteries to other parts of the nail unit. These tiny branches are called **capillaries.** The capillaries give the nail bed its pinkish color. The capillaries carry blood to the epidermis, just below the nail plate. The result is a healthy pink appearance. The capillaries do not reach into the nail plate. Therefore, the nail plate receives no blood or nutrients. Blood is drained away from the nail unit by veins. **Veins** collect blood from the capillaries and return it to the heart. The nail unit has two veins. Each lateral nail fold has its own vein. These veins carry blood and waste products away from the nail bed. Figure 1.5 shows the complex system of veins, arteries, and capillaries found in the hand and finger.

Nerves follow a similar path through the nail unit. Nerves provide the sensations of touch, pain, and warmth. They also move the muscles in the fingers and hands. The nerves end near the skin's surface. The nerve endings are very sensitive. Some are sensitive to pain, some to pressure and others to heat. They relay these sensations back to the brain.

The Hyponychium

The farthest or most distal edge of the nail unit is the **hyponychium.** It is found under the free edge. The hyponychium is composed of epidermis tissue. As you know, this same tissue makes up the top layer of the nail bed (see Figure 1.2).

The hyponychium forms a watertight seal that prevents bacteria, fungi, viruses, etc., from attacking the nail bed. Care should be taken when manicuring under the free edge. Damage to the hyponychium can lead to infection. Once infected, the natural nail plate may lift or separate from the nail bed. It may even lead to loss of the nail plate.

The Onychodermal Band

This feature of the nail unit is often missed. It can only be seen with careful observation. The **onychodermal band** is found in the nail plate, just before the free edge. Examine your own nails for this band. This thin band has a glassy-looking, grayish appearance. You will see this grayish band lying beside the nail plate's white free edge. This is the seal between the nail plate and hyponychium. When this seal is broken, infection often occurs.

The Bone

One of the purposes of the nail plate and bed is to protect the bone in the fingertip. The bone determines the overall shape, curvature, and spread of the nail unit. It also gives strength and support.

In the next chapter, you will learn how various parts of the nail unit work in harmony to grow healthy fingernail plates.

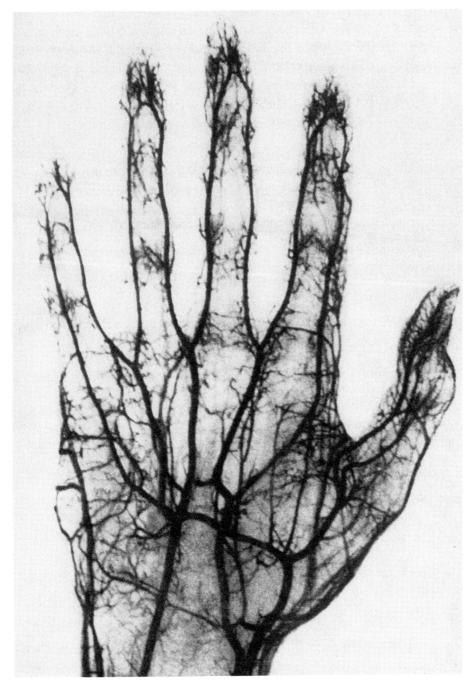

Fig. 1.5
Complex system of veins, arteries, and capillaries found in the hand and fingers. *(Courtesy Creative Nail Design Systems, Inc.)*

■ FAST TRACK

- The fingernail has seven major parts which together form the nail unit.

- The skin fold protecting emerging nail plate is called the *proximal nail fold.*

- Proximal means "nearest attached end."

- The proximal nail fold forms a seal or barrier that protects the nail growth matrix.

- The skin on either side of the nail plate is called the lateral nail fold.

- *Lateral* means "to the side."

- Damage to a nail fold may allow attack by bacteria, fungi, or viruses.

- Below the proximal nail fold is the matrix, the most important part of the nail unit.

- The nail plate grows from special cells in the matrix.

- The matrix's size and shape determines the thickness and width of the nail plate.

- The underside of the proximal nail fold sheds the true cuticle.

- The eponychium is the visible skin fold that appears to end at the nail plate.

- The nail plate is mostly keratin, a protein made from amino acids.

- The part of the nail plate that grows beyond the fingertip is called the free edge, or distal, nail plate.

- Distal means "farthest from the attached end."

- Thinned nail plates cannot properly protect the delicate tissue underneath.

- Overfiling the natural nail is a leading cause of nail plate thinning and destruction.

- Keratin cells leave the matrix looking plump and whitish, but they emerge from under the eponychium flat, transparent, and colorless.

- The lunula is the whitish, opaque area at the base (proximal end) of the nail plate.

- The lunula is formed by cells that have yet to flatten or lose their inner material.

- The thumb with the largest lunula is on the dominant hand.

- The lunula also determines the shape of the nail plate and matches the free edge.

- The nail bed lies directly under the nail plate.

- The nail bed is made of two types of tissue, dermis and epidermis.

- The dermis is the lower or *basement layer* of tissue.

- The epidermis is the upper layer and is closest to the nail plate.

- The dermis has grooves or channels that guide the ridges of the epidermis.

- The dermis is firmly attached to the bone underneath and does not move.

- The epidermis attached to the nail plate and moves with the plate as it grows.

- Epidermis seen on the underside of the free edge is called solehorn or solehorn cuticle.

- Nutrients are delivered to the nail unit by the blood.

- Two arteries supply each nail unit, one runs along each side of the finger.

- Many small branches, called capillaries, carry blood from the arteries to the nail unit.

- The blood in the capillaries give the nail bed its pinkish color.

- The nail plate itself receives no blood or nutrients.

- Blood is drained away from the nail unit by a vein in each lateral nail fold.

- Nerves in the the nail unit provide touch, pain, and warmth sensations.

- Nerves also move the muscles in the fingers and hands.

- The hyponychium is the farthest or most distal edge of the nail unit.

- The hyponychium is composed of the same tissue found in the top layer of the nail bed.

- The hyponychium makes a seal that helps prevents infection of the nail bed.

- Damage to the hyponychium can lead to separation from the nail bed or loss of the nail plate.

- The onychodermal band is a glassy-looking, grayish band found in the nail plate, just before the free edge.

- The onychodermal band is the seal between the nail plate and hyponychium.

- The nail plate and nail bed protect the bone in the fingertip.

- The bone determines the overall shape, curvature, and spread of the nail unit.

- The bone also provides strength and support.

Questions

Chapter 1

1. What is the difference between the proximal, distal and lateral?

2. Why does the little finger have the narrowest nail plate?

3. If a person was born with thin nails, their _____ must be shorter than normal.

4. List ten parts of the nail unit.

5. _____ carry blood and nutrients from the heart to the nail unit while _____ carry blood and waste products away from the nail unit.

6. Name the two types of tissue found in the nail bed and their location.

7. Why is it dangerous to overfile the natural nail plate?

8. What chemical substance is the nail plate composed of and where else on the body is it found?

9. What may happen if the hyponychium is accidentally broken?

10. If the nail plate is firmly attached to the nail bed, how can it move when it grows?

Chapter

T W O

Fingernail Growth and Function

In the last chapter, you learned about the various parts of the nail unit. Now you will see how these parts function. The nail unit is like an orchestra, many instruments working together in concert to create something beautiful. The same is true of the fingernail.

Nail Plate Growth

How fast does the nail plate grow? This is a difficult question to answer. Many factors affect the growth rate. For example, the nail plates of each finger grows at different rates. Nail plates also grow slower at night and during the winter. On the average, the normal thumb nail will grow about $1/10$ inch per month or $1 1/2$ inches per year. The left thumb nail usually grows slightly faster than the right. The index fingernail plate grows the fastest, followed by the pointer and ring finger, which grow at almost the same rate. The thumb's is the next slowest, but the slowest of all is the little finger's. It grows about $1 1/4$ inches per year. As a rule, the longer the finger the faster the nail plate will grow.

Nail plates grow about 20% faster in the summer. They also grow faster during pregnancy. Nail plate growth increases by about $3 1/2$% between the fourth and eighth month of pregnancy. From the ninth month until after delivery, growth rate increases by 20%, regardless of season. After two or three weeks the growth rate drops back to normal. Age also affects the growth rate. Growth peaks between the ages of ten and 14 years and slowly declines after age 20. Nail-biting, accidental damage, or loss causes nail plates to grow faster. Men's nail plates grow faster than women, especially on the dominant hand. Many factors cause slow growth of nail plates. For example, being immobilized or paralyzed, poor circulation, malnutrition, lactation, serious infections, psoriasis, and certain medications.

Some believe that certain foods, (*i.e.,* gelatin or using special creams and oils), will increase the growth rate. This is untrue. Although the nail plate requires certain nutrients for proper growth, there is little evidence that eating any particular foods will cause them to grow faster. Creams, oils, and lotions are sometimes sold as "growth accelerators." These claims are false, misleading, and illegal! No cosmetic product may claim that it will change or alter any body function. These products and other cosmetics are for beautifying only, not healing. Only medical drugs can make such claims. *Remember – no cosmetic-related product can heal, repair, grow, or make any other similar claim.*

The Role of Proper Circulation

In the last chapter, you learned that the matrix is responsible for nail plate growth. Of course, the matrix couldn't perform this task without help. The matrix needs a good blood supply in order to do its job. Arteries carry nutrients to tiny capillaries in the matrix. Capillaries are like long, one-way streets. They wind through tissue carrying blood. The matrix has two types of capillaries. One type delivers oxygen, and important nutrients to matrix cells. The other drains waste products and other contaminant's away from the matrix.

The draining capillaries carry wastes to the veins. The impure blood flows through the kidney and liver where it is purified and returned to the heart. The heart pumps the blood to the arteries which circulates it throughout the body. This cycle runs continuously, 24 hours a day. Every cell in the body benefits from this cycle, including those of the nail unit. This is how the matrix is fed and cleaned. Obviously, proper circulation is a critical part of maintaining a healthy nail unit.

What are Cells?

Each organ in the body is made up of **cells.** The kidney has millions of kidney cells, the heart is made of many heart cells, and so on. In general, biologists define cells as the smallest and simplest units capable of being alive. We are actually a huge colony of cells working together. Our cells are too tiny to be seen by the eye. Most cells in the body are .0004 (four ten-thousandths) of an inch in diameter.

Surprisingly, cells in the nail unit are remarkably similar to other cells like those found in the liver and kidney cells. Even bacteria and plant cells share many common features with cells in our body. All cells bring in food and use it to live and reproduce. They use both oxygen and nutrients then excrete whatever waste is leftover.

The Building Blocks

The matrix is much like the dermis of the skin. Both are made up of special cells that are locked firmly in place. In other words, a matrix cell never becomes part of the nail plate. The matrix cell are like incubators. They grow the cells that eventually become part of the plate. When the plate cells mature they are released from the matrix. As more plate cells are made, the new cells push the older cells toward the eponychium and lunula. This is the process we call "growth of the natural nail."

The plate cells are made of **keratin.** Keratin is a type of protein. Like all protein, keratin is composed of **amino acids.** Amino acids are called the "building blocks of life." They link together in various fashions to make most parts of the body. Amino acids are actually very small chemicals. They are over 13,000 times smaller than a cell. When amino acids are linked together into long strings or chains they are called **proteins.** Therefore, nail plate keratin is a protein made from long chains of amino acids. The same is true for hair and skin.

If hair, skin, and nails all contain keratin, why are they so different? The reason is simple. There are many kinds of amino acids. Different arrangements of amino acids make different types of proteins. Amino acids are like letters of the alphabet. Twenty-six letters can be used to spell an almost unlimited number of words. Since there are more than 20 amino acids, you can see why so many different proteins are found in the body.

Cross-linked for Strength

A protein can be thought of as a long rope made of amino acids. Imagine two ropes laying side by side. If you tie shorter pieces of rope between them you'll make a rope ladder. Tie several rope ladders together and you now have a net! The rope, net, and ladder are all made from the same material, but they are certainly very different.

Protein chains can also be tied together like a rope ladder. The rungs or steps on the protein ladder are called **cross-links.** The cross-links are made from a special type

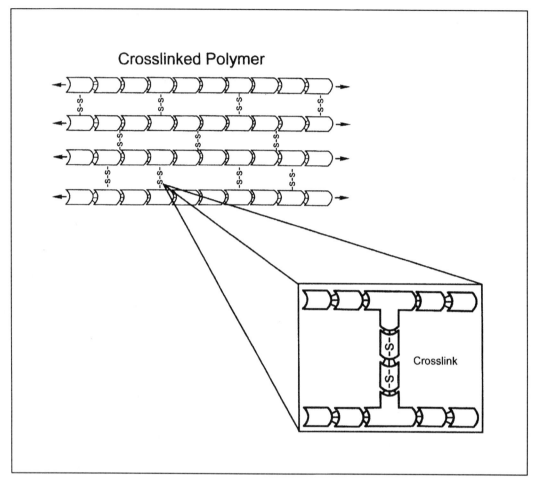

Fig. 2.1
Polymer chain cross-linked with sulfur bonds. *(Courtesy Paul Rollins.)*

of amino acid called **cystine.** Cystine forms the **sulfur cross-links** in hair that make it curly. Very curly hair has many more cross-links than straight hair. In fact, breaking and reforming these sulfur cross-links are the basis for permanent waving procedures. These links are called sulfur cross-links because cystine contains sulfur in its structure. When two cystine lay side by side on a protein chain, the two sulfurs are strongly attracted to each other. They bond and form cross-links between themselves, (Figure 2.1). This attraction or bond is very difficult to break.

The combined strength of millions of sulfur cross-links is what makes nail plates so strong. The natural nail contains much more cystine than hair and skin. As you can imagine, it has many more sulfur cross-links. You will see in later chapters that cross-links are important for other reasons. Some types of advanced, artificial nail enhancements copy nature by using cross-links. This makes the product stronger. Cross-links are a very important concept in nail structure and product chemistry.

How Does the Nail Plate Grow?

As keratin cells are pushed from the matrix they begin to change. They slowly lose their plump, round shape, as shown in Figure 2.2. When they flatten, most of the whitish material inside the cell is lost. They become thin, flat, transparent nail cells. If you recall, the distal part of the matrix is just below the lunula. Most of the lunula area cells haven't completely flattened or lost their inner material. This explains why the lunula is whitish and cloudy. When the cells flatten, they also become more compact. Older cells pack together more tightly making the nail plate harder or more dense, so near the eponychium (proximal nail plate), the plate is softer. The free edge contains the oldest, flattest, and hardest cells.

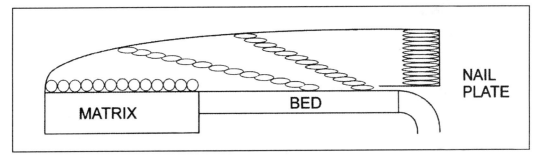

Fig. 2.2
As keratin cells leave the matrix, they begin to flatten and lose their normal, round shape. *(Courtesy Paul Rollins.)*

It is very important to treat the area near the cuticle with care. It is thinner and softer than the rest of the plate. Also, the matrix is directly below this region. Remember, the eponychium tissue is a barrier against bacteria and other microscopic invaders. It must not be broken or harmed. Always use caution with any procedure involving this area of the nail unit. Damage here can permanently injure the nail unit.

For many years, it was believed that at least part of the nail plate grew up from the nail bed. As you learned in Chapter 1, this is incorrect. Every cell in the nail plate comes from the matrix. The only exception is the thin layer of epidermis that adheres to the bottom of the plate. This tissue becomes the solehorn found under the free edge of the plate.

Direction of Growth and Thickness

The matrix cells point at an angle toward the cuticle as shown in Figure 2.3. This creates the flat and thin shape of the plate. The length of the matrix determines the thickness of the natural nail plate. Figure 2.4 shows how this occurs. Clearly, the matrix making the longest row of cells will have the tallest stack of cells in the plate. Of course, a real nail plate has thousands of packed cell layers.

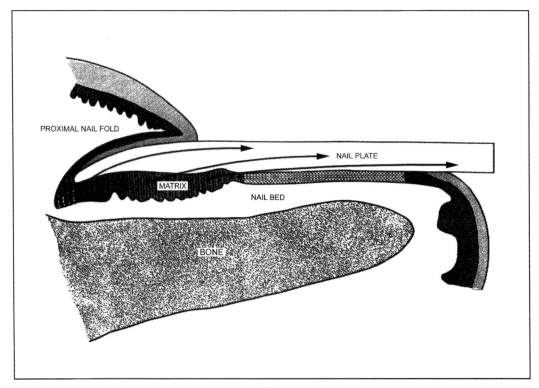

Fig. 2.3
The matrix pushes new keratin cells upward at an angle. The cells in the back of the matrix become the top of the nail plate. Cells pushed from the front of the matrix become the bottom of the nail plate. *(Courtesy Paul Rollins.)*

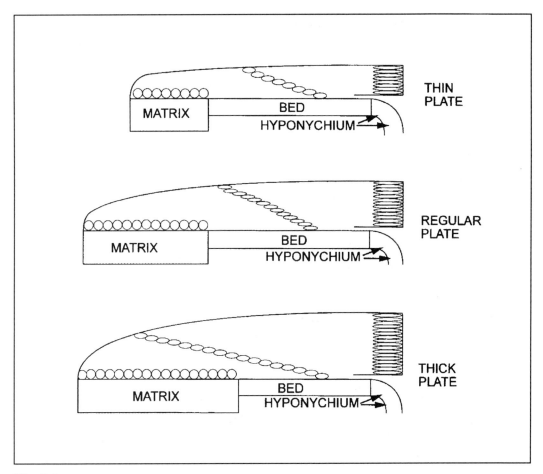

Fig. 2.4
The length of the nail matrix determines nail plate thickness. *(Courtesy Paul Rollins.)*

Look closely at Figure 2.4 and you will see something else interesting about nail plate growth. This diagram shows that the cells near the back of the matrix have much further to travel before they get to the free edge. The cells coming from the back of the matrix end up on top of the plate. Since they travel further, they must be older than cells below them. At the free edge the surface plate cells are nearly two months older than the cells on the bottom side. This may explain why thin, dry nail plates tend to peel at the top surface, rather than from underneath.

What are Strength and Flexibility?

Before we can understand what makes the nails strong and flexible we must define these terms. Strength, hardness, toughness, flexibility, and brittleness are often misused. The following definitions apply to all types of material, not just nail plates.

1. **Strength** is the ability of the nail plate to withstand breakage.

2. **Hardness** measures how easily the plate is scratched or dented.

3. **Flexibility** determines how much the plate will bend.

4. **Brittleness** shows how likely the nail is to break.

5. **Toughness** is a combination of strength and flexibility.

The definitions of these terms are very important to understand. They can be misleading. For example, a product or treatment may claim to "make the nails harder." Most would assume this means the nails would be stronger or more flexible. Such products usually do the opposite, making them stiff and brittle. Why are harder nail plates really less flexible? They are less flexible because they are more brittle. Therefore, brittleness causes nails to be less flexible and have lower strength. So you can see, products that make nail plates harder usually have less strength and lower flexibility. Flexibility is often confused with strength. As you can see from the definition, they are very different. Many things are very flexible, but have no strength. Aluminum can pop-tops are an excellent example. They are very flexible, but bend them a few times and they will snap off.

Chemical Composition of the Nail Plate

Analysis of nail clippings shows that besides amino acids and sulfur, the plate contains many other chemicals. Some of these are iron, aluminum, copper, silver, gold, titanium, phosphorus, zinc, sodium, and calcium. Each of these are found in extremely low concentrations. A common myth is that eating calcium makes nails stronger. This is very unlikely since calcium is only seven one hundredths of a percent (0.07%) of the nail. Sulfur, on the other hand, is about 5% of the nail plate. Sodium is $3^1/2$ times more abundant than calcium in nail plates. Obviously, eating lots of salt (sodium chloride) won't make nails stronger!

What Makes Nails Strong?

Nail plates are a unique combination of strength and flexibility. In other words, the nail is **tough** (see definition for Toughness, above). The nail's strength comes from the many sulfur cross-links and other types of chemical bonds. Much of the flexibility is due to moisture. Increasing moisture content of the nail plate will increase flexibility. The nail plate is not as solid as it seems. If you could shrink to the size of a water molecule you would see that the nail plate was filled with caves and tunnels. These tunnels connect with other tunnels which lead deeper into the plate. They allow water to move freely from the nail bed to the surface of the nail plate.

Even though the plate seems dry, these spaces are filled with moisture. A constant tide of water is flowing upward from the bed through the plate. Once the moisture reaches the surface it evaporates. The moisture acts as a lubricant and a shock absorber. The nail plate is a tangled mass of long keratin strands. Moisture slips between these protein strands. Wet strands slide past each other more easily. The result is higher flexibility. The keratin strands would rather coil up like a loose spring. They can do this more easily if water is present. Protein coiling also increases flexibility. If the plate is suddenly hit or jammed, the water between the keratin chains will also soften the blow. The water absorbs some of the shock. In this way the plate is toughened.

Solvent Effects

Obviously, anything that would remove water or dry out the nail plate would lower flexibility and toughness. Product removers and polish removers contain solvents that can dry the nail plate. Some examples are ethyl acetate and methyl ethyl ketone. These are usually called nonacetone removers. Acetone can remove water from the plate, too. However, normal use of these solvents is unlikely to damage the plate. The drying effect is only temporary.

Why is the drying effect only temporary? Remember, the microscopic tunnels in the nail plate reach all the way to the nail bed. Water is constantly flowing upwards and evaporating from the surface. Any water removed by solvents will be quickly replaced. Some polish removers offset the drying effects by adding up to 20% water. This makes the remover much less drying, but also makes it work a little slower. These removers usually contain special moisturizing agents that help increase flexibility. Normally, only people who constantly have their hands in drying solvents will experience problems. Sometimes people with naturally dry, brittle nail plates may experience peeling or splitting after using drying solvents. If you have a client with dry, flaky nail plates you can dilute polish remover with water yourself. By experimenting, you can find the best ratio of water-to-polish remover. Usually, ten parts polish remover to one or two parts water give the best results.

Splitting, peeling, and breakage can be caused by too much water. People who always have their hands in water often have skin and nail problems (*i.e.,* cosmetologists and frequent hand washers). Excessive water in the nail plates may oversoften the nails. Also, the extra water can cause them to swell. Repeated softening and swelling of the plates may lead to surface peeling. The surface keratin cells are the oldest and easily damaged. Excessive water and drying solvents are most likely to do their harm on the surface.

Creams and lotions can prevent nail plates from drying out. Oily creams can't moisturize by themselves. Only water can moisturize. However, oils sit on top of the nail plate and prevent water evaporation from the surface. This will cause water to build up inside the nail plate and prevent dryness. Oil-based lotions or creams will help clients who have their hands in water all the time. Oils seal the skin and nail plates ,making them water repellent. Detergents also have a negative effect on both nails and skin. They strip away oils that act as softeners and sealers. You will learn more about the skin and how to protect it in Chapter 9.

■ FAST TRACK

- Many factors affect the growth rate of natural nail plates.

- The normal thumbnail will grow an average of $1^1/_2$ inches per year.

- As a rule, the longer the finger the faster the nail plate will grow.

- Age also affects the growth rate. Growth peaks between the ages of ten and 14 years.

- Health factors cause slow growth of nail plates, (*ie.,* being paralyzed, poor circulation, malnutrition, lactation, serious infections, psoriasis, and certain medications).

- Foods, special creams, and oils DO NOT increase the growth rate.

- Creams, oils, and lotions which claim to "accelerate growth" are illegal!

- No cosmetic product may claim that it will change or alter any bodyfunction.

- The nail matrix needs a good blood supply.

- Arteries carry nutrients to tiny capillaries in the matrix.

- Capillaries wind through tissue, carrying blood.

- Their are two types of capillaries; one type delivers oxygen and nutrients, and the second type carries away waste products.

- Each organ in the body is made up of cells.

- Cells are the smallest and simplest units capable of being alive.

- Matrix cells are incubators that grow the cells of the nail plate.

- Plate cells are made of keratin, a protein composed of amino acids.

- Amino acids are called the "building blocks of life."

- Amino acids linked together into long strings or chains are called proteins.

- Nail plate keratin is a protein made from long chains of amino acids.

- Cross-links are made from a special type of amino acid called cystine.

- Cystine forms the sulfur cross-links in hair that make it curly.

- The natural nail contains much more cystine and cross-links than hair and skin.

- As keratin cells leave the matrix they lose their plump, round shape.

- Lunula area cells haven't flattened or lost their inner material.

- The free edge of the plate contains the oldest, flattest, and hard cells.

- The eponychium tissue is a barrier against bacteria and other microscopic invaders.

- Every cell in the nail plate comes from the matrix.

- The length of the matrix determines the thickness of the natural nail plate.

- Strength is the ability of the nail plate to withstand breakage.

- Hardness measures how easily the plate is scratched or dented.

- Flexibility determines how much the plate will bend.

- Brittleness shows how likely the nail is to break.

- Toughness is a combination of strength and flexibility.

- In nail plates the combination of strength and flexibility create toughness.

- Strength comes from the many sulfur cross-links and other types of chemical bonds.

- The nail plate flexibility is created by moisture.

- Product removers and polish removers contain solvents that can dry the nail plate.

- Normal use of these solvents is unlikely to damage the plate.

- Splitting, peeling, and breakage can be caused by too much water.

- Excessive water in the nail plates may oversoften the nails.

- Creams and lotions can prevent nail plates from drying out.

Questions

Chapter 2

1. How fast does a normal thumbnail plate grow in one month? A year?

2. How much slower than the thumb's does the little finger's nail grow in one year?

3. Why is it illegal for cosmetic-related products to claim they "make the nail grow faster"?

4. What are cells?

5. What makes keratin protein stronger than other types of proteins?

6. What part of the nail plate has the oldest cells?

7. Define strength, hardness, flexibility, brittleness, and toughness.

8. Nail plates combine strength and flexibility to make them _____.

9. The nail's strength comes from _____ and other types of chemical bonds. The flexibility is created by _____.

10. Some solvents can _____ the nail plate, but the effect is _____.

THREE

Chemistry Simplified: The Basics

Why do nail technicians need to understand chemistry? Almost every part of the nail technicians job is related to chemistry. Even if you think you just want to "do nails," your success depends on having a good understanding of chemicals and chemistry.

What is a Chemical?

Most people think all chemicals are dangerous, toxic substances. This is completely false! Everything around you is made of chemicals. The walls, this book, food, vitamins, even oxygen is a chemical. In fact, *everything you can see or touch, except light and electricity, is a **chemical.*** Generally, the word "chemical" is only used in a negative way. We forget that just about everything is made of chemicals.

In Chapter 1, we learned that nail plates are 100% chemical. They are mostly protein made from amino acids. Both of these are chemicals. Amino acids are composed of the chemicals, carbon, nitrogen, oxygen, hydrogen, and sulfur. The chemical sulfur is responsible for the sulfur cross-links that make nail plates strong, hair curly, and skin elastic. Nail plates also contain traces of the iron, aluminum, copper, silver, gold, and other chemicals. All matter is made of chemicals.

Matter and Energy

Everything in the world is either matter or energy. **Matter** is anything that takes up space or occupies an area. For instance, books occupy space and cover a measurable area. If the book is 8" × 4" × 2," this is the space it occupies. A book is made of matter. Very few things don't take up space. Even microscopic bacteria use a small amount of space.

Matter can exist in several forms. It can be solid, liquid, or gas. Most matter exist in one or two forms. Some types of matter can exist in all three forms. Water is an excellent example. Water can be frozen into a solid, melted to a liquid, and evaporated into a gas or vapor.

Light, radio waves, microwaves, and Xrays are a few examples of things that don't fill an area. These are not made of matter – they are energy. Energy has no substance and is not made of matter. However, energy can affect matter in many ways. Energy is the only thing that is not made of chemicals.

Molecules

Water is a chemical made from two parts hydrogen and one part oxygen. Chemical shorthand for this combination is H_2O. One molecule of oxygen combined with two molecules of hydrogen makes one molecule of water. A **molecule** is a chemical in its simplest form. If the water molecule were broken down further, it wouldn't be water anymore. It would go back to being molecules of the gases hydrogen and oxygen. Molecules that cannot be broken down any further are called elements. Oxygen and hydrogen are two of the 106 known **elements.** If you could shrink down small enough to see a molecule of water, you would find that a water droplet contains trillions of individual water molecules. These molecules are so small that if a glass of water were enlarged to the size of Earth, the water molecules would only be the size of volleyballs.

Vapors and Fumes

Vapors are a special type of gas. **Vapors** are formed when liquids evaporate into the air. For example, the evaporation of water makes water vapors. Water vapors may be cooled back into the liquid state. Converting a liquid into a gas is called **vaporization.** Some liquids must be heated before they will evaporate. Others will evaporate or **vaporize** at room temperature. Liquids that easily evaporate at room temperature must be kept in closed containers to prevent them from escaping into the air.

Many salon chemicals will easily evaporate. Nail polish is a good example. Some of the polish ingredients will evaporate quickly. This is why nail polish thickens over time. The polish hasn't "gone bad." Instead, some of the ingredients have evaporated away. Obviously, keeping the cap tightly sealed will prevent vapors from escaping. Substances that evaporate easily at room temperature are called **volatile.** Increasing the temperature of a volatile liquid will speed up evaporation. For example, blow dryers evaporate water from hair because the temperature is raised. On hot days, volatile ingredients in salon products will evaporate more quickly, as well. Storing products in a cool location, out of direct sunlight, and closed tightly will keep them in top condition.

Fumes are tiny, solid particles suspended in smoke. Examples of fumes are: car exhaust, smoke from chimneys and welding fumes. Fumes *are not* found in the salon. No salon product releases fumes. This word is frequently misused and should be avoided when talking about salon vapors or odors.

Odors and Vapors

Odors are caused by vapors in the air. These vapors touch sensitive nerves in the nose lining. The nerves send messages to the brain. The messages report the vapor's odor so that the brain can identify it. For example, the nerves may detect chemical vapors from a lemon and send a lemon signal to the brain. The brain determines whether it likes the odor or not and decides what to do.

Our noses are extremely sensitive odor detectors. Even so, every vapor is different. Some vapors are noticeable in very low amounts or concentrations. Other vapors must be highly concentrated before we smell them. Odors can be deceiving. A strong smell can have two different causes:

1. There are a lot of the vapor's molecules in the air.

2. It may also mean that the nerves in the nose are very sensitive to that vapor's molecule, even in extremely low amounts.

Some molecules smell very strong even if there is only one vapor molecule mixed with one million air molecules or one ppm. This is how vapors are measured in the air, in parts of vapor per million parts of air. You will see this written as **ppm** or **parts per million.** For example, 20 vapor molecules in one million molecules of air is 20 ppm. Imagine finding one pink straw in a haystack of over one million yellow straws! This is how sensitive the nose is to some vapors. Since some molecules are more difficult to smell, it is practically impossible for your nose to tell how much vapor is in the air. One chemical may smell strong at two ppm and others smell very weak at 1000 ppm.

When vapors are difficult to smell they are sometimes called **odorless.** Does this mean there are no vapor molecules in the air? Probably not! It merely means that they are difficult to smell. The amount of vapor in the air is not determined by the odor. It is determined by the **evaporation rate.** Quickly evaporating liquids produce large amounts of vapors. Some chemicals used in the salon have offensive odors. Many believe that smelly chemicals must be dangerous. This is quite wrong! A bad smell merely means that your brain does not like the odor. It does not mean the chemical is more toxic or dangerous. You will learn more about vapors and odors, and how to control them, in Chapter 10.

Physical Changes

When water freezes or thaws it undergoes a **physical change.** Only the physical appearance is different, it is still water. When a lump of sugar is crushed into powder or dissolved in water it is physically changed. It is still sugar, but now it has a different appearance. If you evaporate a sugar-water mixture, you will find sugar in the bottom of the container. Of course it is sugar, not something different. In each case, the chemical simply changes form or appearance. It is not chemically altered.

Chemical Changes

Matter can be chemically changed, too. For example, burning sugar produces a black tarry substance. This is an example of a **chemical change,** one chemical changing into a completely different chemical substance. Chemical molecules are like Ttinkertoys.® They can be arranged and rearranged into an almost unlimited number of combinations. Petroleum oil can be chemically converted into vitamin C. Acetone can be changed into water or oxygen. Paper can be made into sugar. The possibilities are endless. In Medieval times, alchemists searched in vain for ways to turn lead into gold. Today, even this is possible.

Chemical Reactions

Molecules like to change. If you give them a reason to change, they usually will. When a molecule changes it is called a **chemical reaction.** Many things can cause chemical reactions. However, a chemical reaction requires energy to make it happen. Most chemical reactions get this energy from heat or light. Heat and light are types of energy. Plants use light energy to cause many chemical reactions in their leaves. These chemical reactions make food for the plant. Cooking uses heat energy to cause chemical reactions in food. Eggs become hard when heated because the egg protein undergoes a chemical reaction. Increasing the temperature usually causes chemical reactions to happen more quickly. This is why food cooks faster at higher temperatures. In general, a chemical reaction will happen twice as fast if the temperature is raised by just 10°F.

A major part of a nail technician's work is to cause chemical reactions to occur on the nail plate. Artificial nail enhancements can use either heat or light energy to create the finished product.

Catalyst

A **catalyst** is a chemical that changes the rate of a chemical reaction. In other words, catalysts make chemical reactions go faster or slower. In nail product chemistry catalysts are used to make reactions happen more quickly. Different chemical reactions require different catalysts. A specific catalyst will usually work for only a few types of chemical reactions, much like a key will open certain locks. That is why so many different catalysts exist. Catalysts are very important chemical tools. Many chemical reactions happen very slowly. For instance, graphite (pencil lead) will slowly change into diamond, but would take many thousands of years. Obviously, a graphite-to-diamond catalyst would be an important invention, if it were ever discovered.

Trillions of chemical reactions occur in our bodies every day. Most of these happen very quickly because of catalysts. Reactions that normally take days, happen in fractions of a second with the right catalyst. Nail technicians also use catalysts in their work. Some chemical reactions used to make overlays and sculptured nails would take several months to happen without the proper catalyst. The role of catalysts in professional nail products will be discussed in Chapter 5.

Solvents and Solutes

A **solvent** is anything that dissolves another substance. Solvents are usually liquid. The substance being dissolved is called a **solute.** As a rule, solutes are solids. However, liquids and gases can be solutes. Water is a very good solvent. In fact, water is called the "Universal Solvent" because it will dissolve more substances than any other solvent. Other examples of safe and powerful solvents are toluene and acetone.

Toluene has been used since the 1930s to dissolve ingredients in nail polish. Toluene keeps nail polish in a liquid form until applied. When the solvent evaporates, the polish dries hard. Studies show that the amount of toluene found in salon air is about 200 times lower than federally established safe levels. Even poorly ventilated salons generally have less than one ppm toluene vapors in the air.

Acetone is frequently used as a polish remover and to dissolve nail enhancements. It is the safest solvent used by nail technicians. When used as a polish remover, acetone dissolves old polish (the solute). Acetone works quickly because it is a good solvent. A poor solvent dissolves solutes very slowly. The better the solvent, the faster it will dissolve the solute. However, sometimes a solvent can be too good! In Chapter 2, you learned that putting small amounts of water in polish remover prevents skin dryness. Why is that? Water is a poor solvent for skin oils and acetone is a good skin oil solvent. Small amounts of water make acetone a slightly poorer solvent. Therefore, it will strip away less skin oil. The more water there is in acetone, the less oil it removes from skin. Water is also a poor solvent for nail polish. Otherwise, hand washing would remove the polish. Putting water in polish remover also makes it a slower polish remover. If you put in too much water, it wouldn't work at all.

Solvents only dissolve a certain amount of solute before they become **saturated.** In other words, the solvent cannot dissolve any more solute. Saturated solvents are very ineffective. Using a saturated solvent is a waste of time and needlessly exposes the client's skin. Always use fresh solvents. Fresh, clean solvents work much faster. Never reuse solvents on the next client. Time is money and reusing solvents is a waste of both!

Warming solvents will also making them faster acting. This is especially true for removing artificial nail enhancements. Most removers require 30 minutes to loosen the product at room temperature. Warming the solvent to 105°F (Jacuzzi® temperature) will shorten the time by ten minutes. Warming solvents should be done with great care. Many solvents are highly flammable! Warm the bottle under hot, running water. Never warm solvents on a stove or microwave oven. Loosen the cap so that pressure doesn't build up in the bottle. Also, cover the dish and hand with a damp cloth while soaking to reduce vapors in the air. The manufacturer of the product you use should be able to provide more safe handling information.

Solvents are usually very volatile. Volatile liquids are more likely to contaminate your breathing air with vapors. They may also increase the risk of accidental fire. Fortunately, solvents are easy to use safely. Remember to always use and dispose of solvents as directed by the manufacturers' instructions and Material Safety Data Sheets (MSDS). In Chapter 8 you will learn more about MSDSs and solvent safety.

Is Acetone Safe?

Why do so many nail technicians avoid acetone? Probably because they have heard one of the many untrue myths about this beneficial substance. What is the truth about acetone? Acetone is one of the most important solvents in the world. Except for water itself, acetone is the safest solvent that nail technicians use!

Myth: I was told that acetone is absorbed through the skin, so it is dangerous.

Many chemicals can be absorbed through the skin. Sometimes this can cause harm, but not always! Skin creams, for example, are designed to penetrate the skin. They are not considered dangerous. Because a chemical is absorbed through the skin, doesn't mean it is unsafe. In the case of acetone, it is almost impossible for dangerous amounts to penetrate the skin. Unless you soak daily in acetone for long periods there is little to fear. This is why acetone is safe to use in salons. It is pretty hard to become overexposed to acetone in the salon.

Myth: Doesn't acetone damage the liver or kidneys and cause cancer?

Acetone does NOT cause cancer. It is not considered to be dangerous to the liver or kidneys either, except in cases of massive overexposure. It is extremely unlikely that this could occur in the salon. Many other industries use large amounts of acetone without serious complication. Nail technicians need not worry about suffering internal injury from acetone.

Myth: It is risky to inhale too much acetone.

It is risky to breathe too much of anything, except oxygen. However, nail technicians use relatively small amounts of acetone. It is practically impossible to breathe too much acetone in the salon.

Myth: The FDA is going to ban acetone.

This is an utterly foolish myth. Acetone is considered to be an extremely safe and useful solvent. The **Food and Drug Administration (FDA)** has never even considered banning this important chemical. This is a common myth about many chemicals in the nail industry. These rumors are almost always spread by uninformed individuals. The FDA rarely bans cosmetic chemicals and no nail products are currently being considered. A chemical must be too dangerous to use safely in the salon before the FDA would consider such a ban. This certainly does not apply to acetone.

Myth: Will acetone dry out and damage the natural nail?

Acetone can absorb some water from the natural nail plate, but so will the nonacetone solvents. However, this is not an important issue. Normal moisture levels are restored quickly. This temporary drying causes no damage to the nail plate. In fact, pure acetone will clean the nail plate and improve product adhesion.

Myth: Nonacetone polish removers are safer.

False! Sadly, many nail technicians choose nonacetone polish and product removers because they believe they are safer. Although nonacetone substitutes can also be used safely, none are safer than acetone. Nonacetone removers usually use either ethyl acetate or methyl ethyl ketone as the solvent. Neither are nearly as safe as acetone.

Rules for Working Safely

There are many rules for working safely. They will be discussed in Chapter 8. Below are a few that will help you work safely with solvents:

- Always work in a well-ventilated area.
- Use a self-closing, metal can to dispose of waste.
- Always keep your hands clean and dry.
- Wear safety glasses to help prevent eye damage.
- Store all flammable substances away from flames and heat.
- Never store flammable products in your car trunk.
- Keep all products tightly closed and out of children's reach.

■ FAST TRACK

- Everything you can see or touch, except light and electricity, is a chemical.
- Everything in the world is either matter or energy.
- Matter is anything that takes up space or occupies an area.
- Energy has no substance and is not made of matter.
- A molecule is a chemical in its simplest form.

- Molecules that cannot be broken down any further are called elements.

- Matter can be solid, liquid, or gas.

- Vapors are formed when liquids evaporate into the air.

- Converting a liquid into a gas is called vaporization.

- Some liquids will evaporate, or vaporize, at room temperature.

- Substances that evaporate easily at room temperature are called volatile.

- Increasing the temperature of a volatile liquid will speed up evaporation.

- Fumes are tiny, solid particles suspended in smoke.

- Fumes *are not* found in the salon.

- Odors are caused by vapors in the air.

- Some molecules are detectable even if there is only one ppm or parts per million.

- Vapors that are difficult to smell are called odorless.

- When water freezes or thaws it undergoes a physical change.

- When a molecule changes its structure it is called a chemical reaction.

- Chemical reactions require energy before they can occur.

- Chemical reactions get energy from heat or light.

- Heat and light are both forms of energy.

- Chemical reactions happen twice as fast if the temperature is raised by 10°F.

- Nail enhancements can use either heat or light energy to create the finished product.

- A catalyst is a chemical that changes the rate of a chemical reaction.

- Trillions of chemical reactions occur in our bodies every day.

- A solvent is anything that dissolves another substance.

- A substance that is dissolved by a solvent is called a solute.

- Water is called the "Universal Solvent."

- Toluene has been safely used since the 1930s to dissolve ingredients in nail polish.

- Acetone is the safest solvent used by nail technicians.

- Warming solvents will also making them faster acting.

- Many solvents are highly flammable!

- Solvents are usually very volatile.

- Volatile liquids are more likely to contaminate your breathing air with vapors.

- Because a chemical is absorbed through the skin doesn't mean it is unsafe.

- Always work in a well-ventilated area.

- Use a self-closing, metal container to dispose of waste.

- Always keep your hands clean and dry.

- Wear safety glasses to help prevent eye damage.

- Store all flammable substances away from flames and heat.

- Never store flammable products in your car trunk.

- Keep all products tightly closed and out of children's reach.

Questions

Chapter 3

1. What is a chemical?

2. What is the difference between matter and energy?

3. What is a molecule?

4. What is the difference between vapors and fumes? Give an example of each.

5. What is the cause of all odors in the salon air?

6. Give two reasons that explain why some vapors smell stronger than others.

7. What is the difference between a chemical reaction and a physical change? Give an example of a physical change.

8. What are catalysts? Why do you think they might be important to nail technicians?

9. Define solvents and solutes.

10. Why is it wasteful to use a saturated solvent?

FOUR

Adhesion and Adhesives

Clients expect value for their money. Services such as nail enhancements must be beautiful and problem free. Service breakdown is a waste of time for both the nail technician and client. Often, the problems are related to improper adhesion. Fortunately, adhesion problems are easily prevented. The key to success is understanding the causes and avoiding the common pitfalls. Do this and you'll make more money, in less time and have happier clients.

Adhesion

Adhesion is a force of nature. It is what makes two surfaces stick together. What causes adhesion? To understand why things stick, we must know something about **surfaces.** A surface can be a solid or liquid. Adhesion is caused when the molecules on one surface are attracted to the molecules on another surface. Paint sticks to wood because it is compatible with the wood's surface. The molecules of paint "like" the molecules on the wood's surface. Therefore, they are attracted toward each other. Wet paint forms a liquid surface. When paint is not compatible with the wood's surface it is repelled. The paint would bead up or refuse to stick.

The Teflon® coating on pans makes a surface that repels food. Putting cooking oil in the pan has the same effect as Teflon.® It prevents food from adhering to the surface of the pan. We can find many examples of one surface repelling another. For instance, wax on a car hood. Wax repels water and causes it to bead up. **Beading** and **streaking** are often seen when a solid surface repels a liquid. Oil, tar, and dirt are also repelled and won't stick to a freshly waxed car. Removing oils and waxes change the nature of the surface. Clean, dry surfaces give better adhesion. A clean surface allows the liquid's molecules to get closer and feel the attractive forces of adhesion. Liquids will not bead up on a clean, compatible surface. Instead, they spread out flat.

You've probably noticed that as the wax wears off the car, the water bead spreads out in a flat sheet. This is called **wetting.** When a liquid spreads out over a clean surface there will be much better adhesion. Why? Because the liquid can cover the surface more thoroughly, penetrate deeper, and hold tighter. Any liquid can "wet" a surface, as long as the liquid and solid surfaces are compatible. **Wetting agents** are special ingredients found in many types of products. Wetting agents make liquid surfaces more compatible. Automatic dishwashing detergents use wetting agents to keep water from beading and spotting glass. Laundry detergents use wetting agents to help the detergent soak deep into the fabric, instead of being repelled by the surface. Wetting agents improve adhesion, too. They do this by making liquids more compatible with solid surfaces.

The small area between two surfaces that are adhered together is called the **adhesive bond.** As long as this bond is intact, the surfaces will not come apart. When two surfaces begin to peel away from each other it is called **delamination.** Properly cleaning the solid surface and proper application techniques will help prevent delamination.

Adhesives

An **adhesive** is a chemical that causes two surfaces to stick together. Adhesives are usually liquids. Adhesives allow incompatible surfaces to be permanently joined together. Scotch® tape is a plastic material coated with a sticky adhesive. Without the adhesive coating, the tape backing would not stick. The sticky adhesive layer acts as a "go-between." It holds the tape backing to other substances. Adhesives are much like an anchor on a ship. One end of the anchor holds the ship, the other end attaches to the ground. Another way to think of adhesives is as double-sided sticky tape. Tape with adhesive on both sides can be sandwiched between two surfaces and will hold the surfaces together.

There are many types of adhesives. There are adhesives for wood, paper, plastics, metal, and glass. Different adhesives are compatible with different surfaces. An adhesive that is compatible with both wood and glass could adhere or hold these materials together. It could also hold together two pieces of wood of two pieces of glass. It could not hold metal and wood together.

Glues

Often times the word glue is incorrectly used to describe nail adhesives. Glue is a type of adhesive that is not useful in salons. **Glues** are made from protein, usually animal. They are made by boiling the animal hides, hooves, and bones. White paper glue is an example of this type of adhesive. Obviously, paper glue is not a suitable adhesive for professional salons. True glues are low in strength and do not adhere well to the nail plate. They also dissolve easily in water. To avoid confusion with these substances, it is best to call nail adhesives by their proper name. Nail technicians use advanced adhesives designed specifically for professional salons. They do not contain protein. Remember, although glues are a type of adhesive, they are not the type used in salons. You will learn more about professional salon adhesives in the following chapters.

Primers

As you know, wetting agents make liquids more compatible with a surface. Is there some way to make solid surfaces more compatible with liquids? The answer is yes. **Primers** make the nail plate more compatible with certain liquids. Metals need primers to be applied to keep paint from peeling from the surfaces. Nail polish base coats are primers, too. Nail polish will resist chipping and peeling if a good base coat is used. Base coats are more compatible with the nail plate. Base coats act as the "go-between" or "anchor." They improve adhesion. Primers are sometimes needed with artificial nail enhancements. They are especially useful if the client has oily skin or ski jump-shaped nails. Primers act like double-sided sticky tape. Primers adhere well, even to oily nail plates.

Figure 4.1 shows how primers work. This simplified drawing shows the chemical groups that make up the nail plate surface. These groups have certain shapes and structures. Primer molecules also have special shapes that match the nail plate. Primers use static electricity-like forces to hold them to the nail surface. These forces are different than static electricity, but they hold the primer just like socks stick together when they come out of the dryer. In much the same way, each primer molecule clings to the nail surface.

The other end of the primer is different. Its shape is not a good match for the nail surface. But, it is a good match for the liquid monomers used to create nail enhancements. Liquid monomers are attracted to this end of the primer molecule. As shown in Figure 4.1, the monomers can match the nail surface, but the attraction is weak.

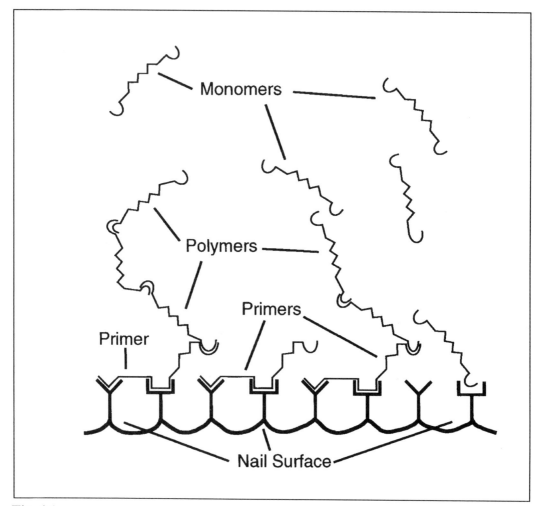

Fig. 4.1
Primers act as "double-sided sticky tape" to anchor monomers firmly to the surface of the natural nail plate. *(Courtesy Paul Rollins.)*

This poor match is why many nail enhancement products need primer. A monomer attaches firmly to the end of a primer, the other end attaches to another monomer. You will see in the next chapter that this is how nail enhancements begin to form.

Primers also remove small molecules of oil that block adhesion. Figure 4.2 shows that oil can lie on the nail surface and prevent good adhesion. Cleansing removes much of the oil, but traces may remain. Primer can dissolve the residual oil and improve adhesion.

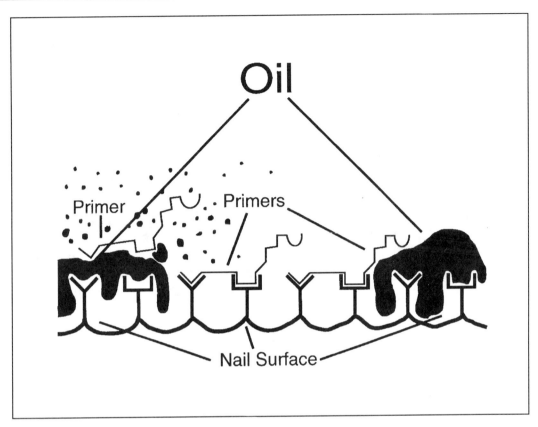

Fig. 4.2
Acid-based primers dissolve molecules of residual oils from the natural nail. These microscopic traces are not removed during normal scrubbing procedures and may lead to service breakdown. *(Courtesy Paul Rollins.)*

Nail primers must be used with caution. Some are very corrosive to skin. A **corrosive** is a substance which can cause visible and sometimes permanent damage to skin. Nail primers, like most professional nail products, should never touch the skin! They can cause painful burns and scars.

A Clean Start

Good adhesion depends on proper technique and high quality products. The best way to ensure success is to start with a clean, dry surface. Scrubbing the nail plate will remove surface oils and other contaminants that interfere with proper adhesion. Many professional nail scrubs will do much more than remove oils. Scrubs get rid of bacteria and fungal spores which lead to infections. Skipping this important step is the major cause of nail infections. It also causes enhancements lifting at the cuticle.

Nail dehydrators are also extremely important. Moisture can interfere with the adhesive bond. This leads to delamination or lifting. To insure proper adhesion always scrub the nail plate, dry thoroughly, and dehydrate. Skipping one step will lead to delamination or lifting. It may also contribute to infections.

Do It Right

Nail products are not all alike. Some are more compatible with the nail plate. Heavy filing may compensate for low quality products and improper application, but it is not the best solution. Of course, if you want to use inferior products or refuse to use proper technique, roughing up the nail may hide your deficiencies. But, it is only a crutch that will eventually lead to failure. Remember, professional products require skill to use correctly. If you are sloppy or use improper application techniques you can expect to have problems. Properly applied, a high quality product doesn't require nail plate abuse.

No Rough Stuff!

One of the most dangerous misconceptions in the professional salon industry is that products don't stick unless you "rough up" the nail. This is absolutely false and very harmful for clients. Nail adhesives work better if the nail plate is clean and dry. Roughing up the nail with heavy abrasives or electric drills is one way to remove oils and dirt, but it is the *wrong way!*

Heavy abrasives strip off much of the natural nail plate, leaving it thin and weak. This leaves no base or supporting structure for the enhancements. When artificial nails are removed, clients quickly discover the damage caused by heavy filing. Some mistakenly believe the products caused the nail to become thin. Actually, it was the nail technician's fault! Rough filing also damages the nail bed. This type of nail bed abuse may cause the nail plate to lift and separate from the nail bed. Once this occurs, clients often develop serious infections under the plate.

Overfiling is a leading cause of nail technician and client problems. It promotes allergic reactions and causes painful burning sensations, infections, loss of the nail plate, product lifting, and breakage. Roughing the plate causes dangerous and excessive thinning of the natural nail. This must be avoided at all cost! It is a myth that product lifting can be prevented by heavy filing. Overfiling is often the cause of lifting and cracking. Thin nail plates are more flexible. There is less nail plate to support the enhancement. The extra flexibility allows the enhancement to bend too easily. This creates invisible, hairline fractures that lead to breakage. The tiny cracks be less than one-quarter the width of a human hair and could go completely unnoticed. However, they will widen and grow longer each time the nail is hit or bumped. Eventually, the cracks will become visible to the client.

Thinning of the nail plate also allows products to soak through the nail plate and into the nail bed. This can cause allergic reactions and chemical burns to the nail bed. Your will learn more about allergic reaction causes and prevention in Chapter 9.

Easy Does It!
Heavy abrasives and high speed drills generate lots of heat. The heat is produced by friction. Rubbing your hands together creates enough heat to make them feel very warm. Imagine how much heat a heavy abrasive or high speed drill can create. This heat can literally burn the nail beds, leaving them sore and damaged. Drills and heavy abrasives can heat the nail bed to over 150°F.

Need to rough up the nail plate to get good adhesion? Then something is wrong! Many nail technicians have great success without rouging up the nail plate. Why? The answer is simple; they properly prepare the nail plates, use correct application techniques, and high quality products. Lifting problems can always be traced back to one of these three areas.

■ FAST TRACK

- Adhesion is a force of nature. It is what makes two surfaces stick together.
- Adhesion is caused when the molecules on one surface are attracted to the molecules on another surface.
- Adhesion occurs when two surfaces are compatible.
- Beading and streaking are often seen when a solid surface repels a liquid.
- Removing oils and waxes change the nature of the surface.
- Clean, dry surfaces give better adhesion.
- Wetting occurs when a liquid and solid surface are compatible.
- Wetting agents make liquid surfaces more compatible.
- The small area between two surfaces that are adhered together is called the adhesive bond.

- When two surfaces begin to peel away from each other it is called delamination.

- An adhesive is a chemical that causes two surfaces to stick together.

- Glues are made from proteins, usually animal.

- Primers are substances that make the nail plate more compatible to certain liquids.

- Good adhesion depends on proper technique and high quality products.

- The best way to ensure success is to start with a clean, dry surface.

- Surface oils and other contaminant's interfere with proper adhesion.

- Moisture can interfere with the adhesive bond.

- Heavy abrasives strip off the natural nail plate, leaving it thin and weak.

- Overfiling is a leading cause of nail technician and client problems.

- Overfiling promotes allergic reactions and causes painful burning sensations, infections, loss of the nail plate, product lifting, and breakage.

- Roughing the plate causes dangerous and excessive thinning of the natural nail.

- Overfiling is often the cause of lifting.

- Thinning of the nail plate can cause allergic reactions and chemical burns to the nail bed.

- Heavy abrasives and high speed drills generate large amounts of heat.

- Drills and heavy abrasives can heat the nail bed to over 150°F.

Questions

Chapter 4

1. What causes adhesion?

2. If two surfaces are not compatible they will _____ each other.

3. _____ are special ingredients that make liquid surfaces more compatible.

4. What is the area between two adhered surfaces called?

5. Define delamination. How is delamination prevented?

6. A(n) _____ is a chemical that causes two surfaces to stick together.

7. Define glue. Why are glues not used in the professional nail industry?

8. Why are nail plate primers used?

9. Is it necessary to "rough up" the nail plate to make high quality, professional nail products adhere well? Explain why.

10. How can drills and heavy abrasives be dangerous?

F I V E

Nail Enhancement Product Chemistry

Many nail technicians know *how* products work, but do they understand *why* they work? "Why" products work is also important. In this chapter you will find that product chemistry is useful and easy to understand.

Fingernail Coatings

As a nail technician, you must perform many tasks. The most important of these is to apply coatings to the nail plate. **Coatings** are products which cover the nail plate with a hard film. Examples of typical coatings are nail polish, topcoats, artificial enhancements, and adhesives.

There are two types of coatings:

    1.   Coatings that cure or polymerize.

    2.   Coatings that harden upon evaporation.

At first these differences may not be obvious, but we'll see that they are like night and day.

Types of Nail Enhancement Coatings

Nail enhancements are a special type of coating used to create artificial fingernails. As you probably know, there are three basic types of nail enhancements.

1. **Natural nail overlays** are coatings which cover only the nail plate.

2. **Tip and overlays** cover an artificial tip and the natural nail plate.

3. Lastly, a **sculptured nail** extends the coating past the free edge of the nailplate to form a tip.

Many different types of products are used to achieve beautiful, artificial nail enhancements. All of these have one thing in common. Every product creates these enhancements by a chemical reaction called **polymerization.**

Monomers and Polymers

In Chapter 3 we learned that a molecule is a chemical in its simplest form. You also learned that molecules are like Tinkertoys.® They can be arranged and rearranged into almost unlimited combinations. Rearranging molecules is called a chemical reaction. Making a nail enhancement is a good example of a chemical reaction. Billions and billions of molecules must react to make just one sculptured nail!

Molecules can hook together into extremely long chains. Each chain contains millions of molecules. Very long chains of molecules are called **polymers.** Polymers can be liquids, but they are usually solid. Polymer comes from two words, **poly** means many and **mer** means units. In this case the "units" are molecules. Therefore, polymers are "many molecules." Chemical reactions that make polymers are called **polymerizations.** Sometimes the term *cure* or *curing* is used, but it has the same meaning.

There are many different types of polymers. Teflon,® nylon, and all plastics are polymers. Even hair and wood are polymers. If you recall from Chapter 2, amino acid molecules linked together into long chains are called proteins. Proteins are also polymers. Nail plates are made of a protein called keratin. So, you can see that nail plates are also polymers.

As you now know, many units (molecules) hook together to make a long polymer chain. By itself, just one of these molecules is called a **monomer. Mono** means one. A monomer is a molecule that makes polymers. The amino acids are monomers that join together to make keratin. At first it may seem a little confusing, but monomers and polymers are the most important words in the nail technician's vocabulary. It is vital that you take the time to acquaint yourself with their meanings.

Understanding Polymerizations

Your clients expect you to be able to solve product-related problems. To do this, you must understand the basics. The answers to many common problems are easy to see, if you understand how monomers cure or **polymerize.** Of course, many types of monomers are used to create nail enhancements. Nail technicians use wraps, liquid-and-powder systems, gels, or no-light gels. Each of these may seem very different, but they are actually quite similar.

The Great Monomers Race

Monomers are like track runners mingling around the starting line, patiently waiting for the race to begin. The race starts when the proper signal is given. Once given, nothing can stop them until they reach the finish line. Monomers also need a signal. This signal starts their race to become polymers. Until that signal is given, they mingle around the container. It takes an **initiator** molecule to give the signal.

An initiator molecule touches a monomer and excites it with a boost of energy. But monomers prefer the quiet life. They don't appreciate too much excitement, so they look for ways to get rid of the extra energy. They do this by attaching themselves to the tail end of another monomer. This passes the extra energy to their new partner. The second monomer doesn't like the energy either, so it uses the same trick. It attaches firmly to a neighboring monomer's tail and passes the energy again. As this game of tag continues, the chain of monomers gets longer and longer. After a while, the growing polymer chains can't find any more monomers. Once the monomer is all gone, the chain reaction stops. We can watch this great race from start to finish while it happens on the nail plate, although monomers are far too small to see. Still, you can observe the effects of their actions.

And They're Off!

Monomers start out as thin liquids or thicker liquids called **gels.** They are free to roam around the container. When the excited initiators begin the reaction, monomer chains sprout up everywhere. They begin to grow longer and longer. Soon, the many long strings of monomers start getting in each other's way. They become tangled and knotted, which makes the product get much thicker. Eventually, the chains are too long to move freely. The product is now a teeming mass of microscopic strings. The polymer is formed, but the chemical reaction is not finished. The surface may be hard enough to file, but it will be days before the chains reach their ultimate lengths.

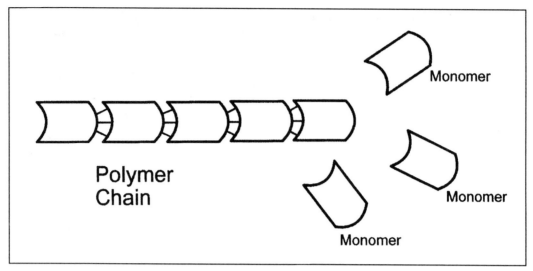

Fig. 5.1
A simple polymer chain grows in one direction by adding monomers in a
head-to-tail fashion. *(Courtesy Paul Rollins.)*

Simple versus Cross-linking

Normally, the head of one monomer reacts with the tail of another, etc. The result
is a long chain of monomers attached head to tail (Figure 5.1). These are called
simple polymer chains. For nail enhancements, these simple polymer chains have
some disadvantages. The tangled chains are easily unraveled by solvents. Recall
from Chapter 3 that a solvent is anything which dissolves another substance. When
the chains unravel, the polymer breaks apart and dissolves. This makes removal
quick and easy. Unfortunately, nail polish removers are solvents which can weaken
some nail enhancement products. The solvents create microscopic cracks. These
may later lead to breakage. Figure 5.2 shows a highly magnified photograph of a
crack caused by solvents. This crack is $1/10$ the thickness of a human hair. Even
though it is small, it can quickly grow larger if hit or stressed. Even a sudden change
in temperature can enlarge it.

Polymer chains can also be unraveled by force. Products with simple polymer
chains are easily damaged by sharp impacts or stresses. Dyes and stains can also get
lodged between the tangled chains. Nail polishes, marker ink, foods, and many
other things can cause unsightly stains on the surface.

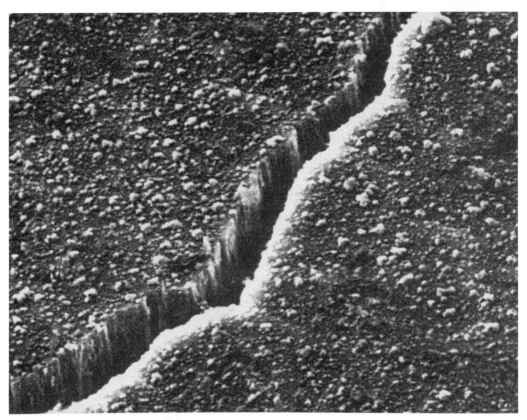

Fig. 5.2
Highly magnified microscopic crack in the surface of a polymer. This crack is
approximately ten microns wide or $^1/_{10}$ the thickness of a human hair.
(Courtesy Creative Nail Design Systems, Inc.)

To overcome these problems, some products use special types of monomers called
cross-linkers. A **cross-linker** is a monomer that can join different polymer chains
together. Cross-linkers are monomers with arms. Normal monomers can join only
head to tail. Cross-linkers also join head to tail, but their extra arms grow new
chains. They also join with other nearby chains. Some cross-linkers can link three
or more chains. Each place where a monomer connects with another chain is called
a **cross-link.** Cross-links are like rungs on a ladder. Cross-links create strong net-
like structures. Cross-links can also join many other layers of cross-linked nets. The
result is a three-dimensional structure of great strength and flexibility. This is how
many types of artificial nail enhancements are made.

Shrinkage

All polymers shrink when they form; there are no exceptions, in any nail product. Monomers are so small that they are invisible even under the most powerful microscope. Still, scientists know many things about monomers. They know that monomers normally don't touch each other. They bounce around the container at high speeds trying to avoid other monomers. They join only when the conditions are right. When they do join, the monomers embrace each other tightly. This explains why polymers shrink. How? Imagine billions of monomers suddenly coming closer together. The effect is very noticeable. In fact, nail enhancement polymers shrink between 3-20%. Some shrink more than others. Excessive shrinkage (above 12%) causes many problems, such as lifting, tip cracking, and other types of service breakdown.

Over cross-linking causes excessive shrinkage, too. Tightly woven nets shrink more than loose weaves. The effects of shrinkage can usually be seen. Too much shrinkage may cause product to lift in the center of the nail plate. When small areas pull away from the nail plate they often look like bubbles. These are caused by excessive shrinkage. As mentioned below, one way to increase the strength without increasing shrinkage is with IPNs. Because IPNs don't add extra cross-links to the net, they create less shrinkage. Another way to control shrinkage is by following manufacturers' directions. Improperly mixing (*i.e.,* too wet a consistency) and incorrect curing polymers may cause excessive shrinkage and other more serious problems. This will be discussed further in later chapters.

In Chapter 2, you learned that the nail plate has sulfur cross-links that create a tough, resilient structure. Obviously, a net is stronger than a single chain. Nets are less likely to break under sudden impacts or stresses. Besides increased strength, the cross-linked nets prevent nail polish, inks, and dyes from staining the surface. They are impervious to nail polish removers, as well. However, they are more resistant to all solvents, so removal is much more difficult.

IPNs

Polymer chains can be strengthened in many ways. Cross-linking is one important way. Unfortunately, a polymer with too much cross-linking is brittle and easily shattered. Too much cross-linking lowers the nail enhancement's flexibility and reduces toughness. However, cross-linked polymers can be made stronger with **IPNs** (short for Interpenetrating Polymer Network). Imagine weaving a strong polymer rope through the holes of the cross-linked net. The rope will add strength to the net without causing brittleness. This is how IPNs work. They start as monomers, but they weave new and different chains through the polymer net. They do not become part of the cross-linked net; instead, they reinforce it! IPNs were first used for high-tech aerospace polymers, but now they are finding their way into the nail industry. Why? Remember from Chapter 2, a balance of strength and flexibility equals toughness. This technology is used to create nail enhancements with dramatically increased strength without sacrificing flexibility.

Energize Me!

Energy is the final key to understanding how monomers become polymers. All monomers need energy to make polymers. You learned that they get this energy from the initiator molecule. Initiator molecules control everything. They are the starting gun that begins the monomer marathon. But where does the initiator molecule get this energy? What is the source? These are some of the most important questions in nail technology.

Different initiators use different kinds of energy. Initiators absorb and hold energy. In a sense, they are like batteries. Some initiators only absorb light energy. Other initiators only absorb heat energy. Light and heat are the only energy useful for making nail enhancement polymers. Products that require light generally use ultraviolet light. All other products use heat energy.

Light and Heat Energy

If you have ever seen sunlight passing through a prism or seen a rainbow in the sky you know that sunlight is made of many colors. These colors are called the **visible spectrum.** Each of these colors are actually energy. Solar cells turn light energy into electricity. Clearly, light is a powerful form of energy.

Each color we see is a different level of energy. That is why they look different to our eyes. Red is the lowest energy level of visible light. Violet is the highest energy level of visible light. Most other energy levels are either too strong or too weak to see. For example, the next energy level above violet is called **ultraviolet light** or **UV light.** We cannot see UV light, but we do see its effects. UV light tans the skin. Light energy just below the color red is called **infrared light**. We can't see infrared light, but we feel it. Infrared light is also called heat. **Heat** is a form of light that we cannot see. Its energy level is too low. But unlike our eyes, the skin is sensitive to infrared light energy.

Don't Watch That UV-A Exposure

There are three types of ultraviolet light. They are UV-A, UV-B, and UV-C. All three are found in sunlight. Overexposure to UV-B and UV-C is dangerous to skin and eyes. They cause premature wrinkling of the skin, eye damage, and certain types of skin cancers. UV-A is far safer, but it is not risk free. It is far less likely to cause harm. Of course, you can't be harmed unless you are overexposed. Even overexposure to heat (infrared light) can be damaging. In short, UV-A exposure is safe unless overexposure occurs. The amount of UV-A used to cure artificial nail enhancements is very low. Your client will get more UV light exposure when they drive home on a sunny day! The only precautions needed are for the nail technicians: Always place the lamp so that you cannot see directly into the lit chamber.

Understanding which type of energy an enhancement product needs can solve many problems. For example, you can see why it is important to cover UV light-curing products even when they are not near a UV gel lamp. Sunlight and even artificial room lights can start polymerization in the container. Also, you can understand why it would be silly to put a heat-curing monomer in a hot car trunk, a store window or some other warm area. The high heat may also cause polymerization in the container. Solving and avoiding problems is easy – if you understand the basics.

Product Type

It is simple to determine the type of energy a product uses. Products that use a special lamp always use light energy. These are called **light-curing products.** All other nail enhancement products use heat. These are called **heat-curing products.** Why don't you have to heat them? The answer is simple. They use the heat in the room and body heat to cause polymerization or curing.

You might not notice the heat in most rooms, unless you had just come in from a snowstorm. Still, there is a tremendous amount of heat in the average room. Otherwise, we would freeze to death. Many monomers cure at room temperature, 68°-74°F. Tip adhesives (also monomers) and wraps are examples. A few products require normal incandescent light bulbs. These are not light-curing monomers. They are using the extra heat released from the light bulb. These products are still heat curing.

Visible Light Cure

Not all light curing products use UV light. Some have initiators that absorb visible light. As you know, violet light is just below ultraviolet in energy. Below violet is blue light. It is possible to cure monomers with violet and blue light. These products have some important advantages, but there is one major draw back. The amount of UV light in the normal salon is very low, except near a sunlit window. There is lots of blue and violet light in a normal room. Just like photographic film, visible light-curing products are highly sensitive to room light. They polymerize much faster than UV-curing products when exposed to normal room lighting. Too much light exposure can cause product thickening and lead to many other problems. Therefore, if you use a visible light-curing product, make certain to minimize exposure to all light. You can easily tell if a product uses visible light. The lights are much brighter and usually very warm. They also produce a white light instead of the familiar purple light of a UV gel lamp.

Catalysts

Although catalysts were discussed in Chapter 3, their role in product chemistry was left until now. As you recall, catalysts are used in nail products to make chemical reactions happen faster. At the beginning of this chapter, initiators were compared to a starting gun. In some ways, catalysts are like the trigger on the gun. Some initiators are very slow and take their time exciting molecules. Catalysts make it easier for the initiator to do its job. They make initiators work faster and more efficiently. Later, you will see that monomers need all three parts; initiator, energy, and catalyst. If one of these is missing, chemical reactions happen much more slowly or not at all.

Exothermic Reactions

When two monomers join, an extremely small amount of heat is released. This is called an **exothermic reaction. Exothermic** means heat releasing. This happens with all types of nail enhancement products. However, some types release more heat than others. Of course, you cannot feel the heat released from two monomers. But remember, it takes many billions of monomers to make a nail enhancement. Can you feel the heat of this many monomers? The answer is definitely yes! This heat is called an **exotherm.** Under certain circumstances it can be quite noticeable, especially for monomers used to make wraps and light-cure products.

Unless the heat causes your clients to become uncomfortable, you should not be overly concerned. Heat-curing products will benefit from the additional energy. It will result in a better enhancement. However, exotherms that burn clients' nail beds can cause damage to the tissue and weaken the enhancement. Since all monomers release heat, why are some more noticeable than others? There are several reasons. Mostly, it depends on how quickly heat is released. Products that release heat very quickly will feel warmer. Products that release heat slowly do not feel warm. In other words, rapid heat buildup is the problem. Below are some other factors that may cause a client to feel an exotherm.

1. Temperature of the room and/or product

The warmer the monomer, the faster it will cure. You learned in Chapter 3 that a 10°F increase makes chemical reactions happen twice as fast. If the room is too warm or the table lamp is above 60 watts, the extra heat makes monomers react faster. Sometimes, your clients will feel their nail beds become very warm, even hot!

Solution: Use low-wattage or cool-fluorescent bulbs and don't store monomers in warm locations. Never put any type of professional nail product in a window, car trunk, or other warm locations. Keep them cool, but not cold.

2. Excessive initiator or catalyst

Faster is not always better. It takes time to do things right. To meet the demands of the nail professional, some manufacturers increase the level of initiator or catalysts to make products cure faster. Faster set means more heat in a shorter time. This can lead to uncomfortably warm exotherms. It also may cause enhancements to lose some flexibility and lower toughness. Wrap catalysts may require that they be sprayed from as far as 12 inches. This prevents too much catalyst from getting on the monomer and causing painful exotherm. The exotherm can reach in excess of 170°F! Luckily, new lower-exothem catalysts are being sold. There are also specially formulated wrap products that don't require an additional catalyst. However, they cure much more slowly.

Solution: Avoid using "fast-set" products that cause clients to feel uncomfortable exotherms. This applies to light-cure products as well. Switch to low-exotherm wrap catalysts or those that require no catalyst.

3. Unhealthy or damaged nail beds

This may be the leading reason for clients' complaints of burning sensations. Damaged nail beds are like a sore tooth. Tapping your finger on a normal tooth doesn't hurt, but don't try it on an aching tooth! Damaged nail beds are very sensitive to heat. Even tiny exotherms are easily felt on these overly sensitive tissues.

Generally, the primary reason for unhealthy nail beds is overfiling and overpriming. Overfiling, usually called "roughing up the nail plate," strips away much of the natural nail. The heat created from heavy abrasives and filing can burn nail beds, leaving them sore and tender. Large-grit files and high-speed drills are usually the culprits. Both can be very damaging to the nail plate and bed. Drill bits use friction to cut away the surface. Friction makes heat and lots of it! But even light abrasive files and drill bits can cause nail bed damage. Filing too hard, too often, or for too long makes nail beds sore and sensitive.

Excessive amounts of nail primers, especially on thinned nail plates, can seep through to the sensitive nail bed tissues and cause further damage. If your client is experiencing painful exotherms it could be that their nails have been abused by overfiling and excessive priming. When it comes to filing and primers, remember— a little goes a long way.

Solution: Use light abrasives and remove the shine, *not the nail.* Filing should only remove oils. Oils are what makes the nail plates shiny and cause products to lift. Don't use the heavy-handed approach when filing. Be gentle with nail plates. Filing too often or with drills can damage a nail bed, too. Also, avoid using too much primer. All that is needed is enough to barely wet the nail plate.

4. Metal sculpting forms

Metal can act as a catalyst. Sculpting on metal forms may cause an extra exotherm, but rarely will it cause burning. Healthy nail beds will experience minimal warming only. As mentioned before, this warming can actually be beneficial to the enhancement.

Solution: Usually no special action is required, since the exotherm is quite mild and beneficial. However, if your client complains, try switching to a nonmetal form.

Evaporation Coatings

Nail polishes, topcoats, and base coats also form coatings on the nail plate. However, these products are entirely different. They do not polymerize. They contain no monomers. These products work strictly by evaporation. The majority of the ingredients are volatile or quickly evaporating solvents (see Chapter 3). Special polymers are dissolved in the solvents. The polymers in these products are not cross-linked polymers so they dissolve easily. As the solvents evaporate, a smooth polymer film is left behind. Artist paints and hair sprays work in the same fashion.

Of course, the strength of uncross-linked polymers is much lower than cross-linked enhancement polymers. This explains why polishes are prone to chipping and are so easily dissolved by removers. Now you can see for yourself the great difference between coatings that cure or polymerize and those that harden upon evaporation. Later, you will learn more about the many other ingredients used in nail polishes, their usefulness, and safety.

Yellowing, Brittleness, and Other Signs of Aging

Yellowing and premature aging of nail enhancements can be caused by many things. Depending on product type, there are several reasons why polymers become dingy or off-colored. Some technicians assume that yellowing or brittleness can't be helped. This is untrue. If an enhancement becomes brittle or off-color, something is wrong. When properly applied, high-quality products do not have these problems. Don't be satisfied with your work until you can create color-stable, strong, and flexible nail enhancements. Below, you will find a list of the most common reasons for these problems. Use this information to avoid these common pitfalls.

1. Uncross-linked simple polymers, such as wraps, can absorb color between the polymer chains causing them to become stained. It can also happen to other types of enhancements if they have too few cross-links. Nail polish and household cleaning products are often the cause. This type of discoloration usually takes time to occur. The freshly applied enhancement must first be exposed to the staining agent. It is usually noticed when the nail polish is removed.

Solution: Always use a base coat to seal the product before applying polish, and wear gloves when cleaning or gardening. You might also consider using products that are cross-linked.

2. Sometimes, nail enhancements discolor immediately upon application. Often times this is a sign of contamination. Brush contamination is usually the cause. Many nail technicians store their brushes upside down (hairs up). Monomer may run into the base of the brush. There it can mix with old monomer and become discolored. If your brush has a wooden handle, contact with the wood can also discolor the monomer. When you flip the brush over to use it, contaminated monomer can then flow down the hairs and cause yellowing. If you use more than one type of product it is wise to use one brush for each product. Contamination can occur when a brush is used with many different products. Once one brush goes into one product, it should never be exposed to another.

Solution: Always lay brushes flat when not in use. The brush's hairs should never touch ANYTHING except your product, a clean wiping towel, and the clients' nail plates. Have a brush for each product you use and never interchange them.

3. Improperly cleaning brushes can also contaminate them. Residues from detergents and oils may cause discoloration and lifting. Liquid monomer users should clean the brush with the monomer. Never use any soap or detergent. Avoid using solvents. They can dry out the hairs over time. They can also get into the handle and allow contaminates to leach into the brush. Gel users must use solvent brush cleaners, but take care. Wipe the brush with a clean paper towel or cloth, swirl in fresh acetone, wipe again, swirl in acetone, then allow brush to air dry in a clean, dark location.

Solution: Value and properly maintain your tools. Clean brushes correctly and never use soaps, detergents, or oils.

4. Products themselves can also become contaminated. A likely source is the dappen dish. Filings and dust can settle in the dappen dish and cause the monomer to partially polymerize, making a gooey gel-like substance. Monomer left in the dappen dish overnight will certainly cause problems, especially if you refill the dish without properly cleaning it first. Pour out only as much monomer as you need. *Never pour monomer back into the container.* You are asking for trouble if you do. A small amount of contaminated monomer can ruin an entire bottle. Use the extra monomer to clean your brush. The extra monomer can then be mixed with small amount of polymer powder and disposed of after it hardens.

Solution: Never pour used product back into the original container. Clean dappen dishes several times each day. Never let liquid monomer sit overnight in a dappen dish.

5. Some products require mixing a small amount of liquid monomer with powdered polymer. These two-part systems are usually called liquid-and-powder systems. Mixing these in the proper ratio or consistency is critical. Too much liquid or powder can have disastrous consequences. Yellowing and brittleness is one effect of improper consistency.

Solution: Be sure you are using the exact consistency recommended by the manufacturer. This is usually a medium-wet bead consistency. More information on this extremely important topic will be given in the next chapter.

6. Many problems, including yellowing and brittleness, can be traced back to incorrect use. Nail technicians often fail to realize the importance of exactly following manufacturer's instructions. A good example is with two-part liquid-and-powder systems. NEVER use one manufacturer's liquid with another manufacturer's powder. Also, NEVER blend together different manufacturer's powders or liquid monomers to make a "custom" product. Doing either of these is foolish, irresponsible, and legally negligent. It is one of the leading causes of allergic reactions in our industry. If the client develops a serious problem, you are legally responsible for your actions. It will be difficult to explain why you did not follow directions. Even the manufacturer of the products will be unable to defend you.

Solution: Follow all instructions exactly. Never mix or break apart systems intended to be used together. Never alter manufacturers' products by mixing or adding other ingredients. If you do, you might have to explain your actions in a court of law.

7. Topcoats are very useful products, but they contain ingredients that can yellow. If you apply them directly over nail enhancements, with time they could become discolored. Usually, once removed, the discoloration disappears.

Solution: Use care when putting topcoat over unpolished nail enhancements. You may wish to avoid their use on clients who are frequently in the sun or use tanning beds.

8. If enhancements become yellow or brittle after several days or weeks, sunlight and air are often the cause. UV light from the sun or tanning bed can quickly discolor enhancements. Ozone (a natural form of oxygen) can also create brittleness. UV light and ozone are responsible for cracks in car dashboards. Sunlight contains so much UV light that it can yellow newspaper in one afternoon. Proper application and product formulation determines a nail enhancement's resistance to these environmental factors.

Product formulation can also lead to yellowing. Properly formulated products are highly resistant to yellowing and premature aging. You will learn later that some products use special absorbers to filter out damaging UV light. Fast-setting liquid-and-powder systems usually yellow and become brittle because of the excessive catalyst or initiator. All products are not the same. They often contain different ingredients or special additives. In general, a poor choice of ingredients create poor products that discolor and become brittle. As the old saying goes, "You get what you pay for." If you use the most inexpensive products, you can't expect them to perform like more-expensive products.

Solution: Ask the product's manufacturer how to prevent enhancement yellowing, and give them a chance to solve your problem. If nothing they suggest seems to work, review your technique and make sure it is correct, from beginning to end. Then, try another product, but remember, if your technique is the problem changing products won't help. To test a new product for resistance to yellowing try the following:

- Adhere several tips to wooden pusher sticks.

- Use these to make an overlay or sculptured nail enhancement as you would usually do.

(Be sure to use a clear powder. Pink powders can cover up product discoloration.) On one tip use your old product. Place the new product on a different tip.

- Place both enhancements in direct sunlight for a few days.

- Check them each day to see which yellows first. (A properly formulated product will not yellow, even after days of exposure.)

- Repeat the test if you are still unsure. Test many products until you find the one you like.

Nail Polish Chemistry

Modern nail polish has been in use since the 1920s. Many things have changed since the original products, but the basic chemistry remains the same. A typical formulation for nail polish consists of four major types of ingredients. Below is a chart which shows these ingredients and following is an explanation of why they are used.

Type of Substance	Chemical Name	Use
Polymer	Nitrocellulose	10%
Polymer	TSF Resin	10%
Plasticizer	Dibutyl Phthalate	5%
Solvent	Ethyl Alcohol	5%
Solvent	Ethyl Acetate	20%
Solvent	Butyl Acetate	15%
Solvent	Toluene	30%
Pigments	Various Colors	0.5%

TSF resin is used to improve adhesion and toughen the polish coating. TSF resin sticks strongly to the nail plate, but it is too soft and dull looking. Nitrocellulose produces very hard shiny surfaces, but does not stick to the nail plate and is too brittle. TSF resin and nitrocellulose make a great pair. TSF resin softens and toughens the nitrocellulose, while improving adhesion. Nitrocellulose strengthens TSF resin and makes it hard and shiny.

Suspension agents are added to make the product easier to use. They are usually finely ground clays. These agents keep the pigments suspended for longer and reduce mixing time. The pigments are the heart of the polish. They provide the color and covering power. A white pigment called titanium dioxide is frequently combined with colored pigments to reduce the number of coats. When combined with color pigments, titanium dioxide produces brilliant long-lasting colors.

Plasticizers increase flexibility and wear of the polymer base. As the name suggests, plasticizers make the polymer more plastic-like by softening it and allowing the coating to give a little under stress. Nail polish polymers by themselves are too brittle and quickly crack or chip. The proper blend of plasticizer and polymer produces a tough film which holds the pigments tightly to the nail plate.

Solvents are needed to make spreadable liquids. They keep the polymer and additives dissolved. After the polish is applied, the solvent evaporates slowly leaving remaining ingredients.

With this background, it is easy to understand why polishes behave differently. If the formulation has too little plasticizer or too much nitrocellulose the film is brittle. Too little TSF resin and the polish will chip and peel away. Polishes that require too many coats to cover completely contain too little titanium dioxide or other pigments. If a polish gets bubbles easily or forms an uneven surface upon drying, usually the reason is a solvent that evaporates too quickly. This effect is seen often times during periods of high temperatures and humidity.

Contains No Formaldehyde

This claim is seen on some nail enamels or polishes. Should formaldehyde be a concern for nail enamel users? In most cases, no! The negligible amount found in enamel is extremely safe. One exception is the prolonged use of products with more than 1% formaldehyde. At these levels, formaldehyde may cause severe allergic reactions.

Nail hardeners may legally contain as much as 3% formaldehyde. Concentrations above 1% will cause the natural nail to stiffen and lose flexibility. Clients usually confuse this stiffening effect with strengthening. They incorrectly assume that harder nails must be stronger. Although the nail bends less, it is actually *losing* strength. In this case, prolonged use of formaldehyde causes the nails to become split, dry and brittle.

Fortunately, most nail enamels contain less than 0.0015% formaldehyde (fifteen ten-thousandths of a percent). This tiny amount comes from an important ingredient called toluene sulfonamide formaldehyde resin (TSF resin). This resin is very different from formaldehyde. Luckily, the traces of formaldehyde will not cause problems unless the client is already allergic to formaldehyde, *i.e.,* from use of formaldehyde nail hardeners.

The only way to eliminate this tiny amount of formaldehyde is to use an inferior resin. Put another way, superior nail enamel formulations contain almost no detectable amounts of formaldehyde. The only reason for using the inferior resin is simply to make the "no-formaldehyde" claim. Obviously, these products offer little benefit for the user, except for the rare client that is allergic to formaldehyde.

Toluene-Free

Toluene has been safely used in nail enamels since the 1930s. In the 1990s toluene has become a very controversial ingredient. Paranoid politicians passed a state law in California that basically says that *safe is not safe enough*. The California law requires exposure to be thousands of times below the federal safe-exposure level. Because of a lawsuit, the State of California asked for a study which would determine the level of toluene in the average salon. This study showed that the toluene found in salon air is more than 200 times below the federal safe limits. In other words, the air would still be safe to breathe even if the toluene vapors of *200* salons were put into one salon.

Toluene is used to dissolve other ingredients in nail enamels. Polishes with toluene apply smoother and produce more brilliant colors that resist peeling. No other solvent does as good a job as toluene. Toluene-containing enamels are clearly superior. Before the results of the California salon study was completed, retail polish manufacturers settled out of court, promising to never use toluene again. The California salon study turned out to be a tremendous break for salons. Now, only professional nail polishes are allowed to use toluene. This means that if clients want superior nail polish, they must buy it from a salon. Otherwise, they can only purchase inferior, toluene-free retail products.

There is little reason to believe that toluene in nail polish is harmful to breathe. However, a 1988 study claimed that toluene causes the natural nail to peel and split.

This effect was seen when nail clippings were soaked for three days in toluene and then examined under a high-power microscope. Obviously, no one would soak their nails in toluene for this long. Therefore, toluene is probably safe for healthy nails. Of course, if your client already has nails that peel or split, it might be wise to avoid toluene-containing products.

TSF Resin

Toluene sulfonamide formaldehyde resin is a polymer produced from each of the chemicals in its name. This particular polymer is widely used to increase the strength of the primary nail polish polymer, nitrocellulose. Hypoallergenic polishes usually contain a polyester resin which makes the polish about 10-20% less durable. Another alternative is toluene sulfonamide epoxy resin. This polymer has slightly better properties than the polyesters. However, polishes which contain this resin suffer from poor shelf life. Neither can it compare to TSF resin for strength and durability.

Base Coats and Topcoats

Base coats and topcoats are formulated with many of the same ingredients as polish. Most base coats contain a high percentage of TSF resin to improve nail plate adhesion. Topcoats generally have high amounts of the nitrocellulose polymer with extra plasticizer and no pigments. This blend will improve strength by thickening the coating and increase the gloss. Still, the way a polish dries has a great deal to do with the final results.

Waiting for a polish to dry is tiresome, but the slower it dries the better! Slower-evaporating solvents produce brighter colors. If a polish is forced to dry quickly by heat or chemical dryers it will usually result in more shrinkage and cracking. Formulations that use rapidly evaporating solvents tend to bubble and pit more or produce uneven surfaces. Blowing on the polish will lower adhesion and gloss. The best results will be obtained by using a base coat, two coats of polish, and a topcoat on a properly prepared nail plate. Pausing as long as you can between each coat will produce a smoother, more brilliant surface. Applying the second coat of polish too quickly is a major reason for the "orange peel" texture effect you may have experienced. This is especially pronounced in times of high temperatures and humidity.

■ FAST TRACK

- ■ Coatings are products which cover the nail plate with a hard film.

- ■ Natural nail overlays are coatings which cover only the nail plate.

- ■ Tip and overlays cover an artificial tip and the natural nail plate.

- ■ A sculptured nail extends the coating past the free edge of the nailplate to form a tip.

- ■ Billions of molecules must react to make just one sculptured nail.

- ■ Very long chains of molecules are called polymers.

- ■ *Poly* means many and *mer* means units.

- ■ Chemical reactions that make polymers are called polymerizations.

- ■ A monomer is a molecule that makes polymers.

- ■ An initiator molecule starts polymerizations.

- ■ Monomers start out as thin liquids, or thicker liquids, called gels.

- ■ Solvents unravel polymer chains, causing them to dissolve.

- ■ Solvents create microscopic cracks that may lead to breakage.

- ■ Cross-linkers are monomers that join different polymer chains together.

- ■ Each place where a monomer connects with another chain is called a cross-link.

- ■ Cross-links create strong net-like structures of great strength and flexibility.

- ■ Cross-linked nets prevent nail polish, inks, and dyes from staining enhancements.

- ■ Cross-linked polymers can be made stronger with an interpenetrating polymer network.

- ■ Sunlight is made of many colors, called the visible spectrum.

- ■ Each color we see is a different level of energy.

- ■ Red is the lowest energy level of visible light.

- ■ Violet is the highest energy level of visible light.

- The next energy level above violet is called ultraviolet light or UV light.

- Light energy just below the color red is called infrared light or heat.

- Products that use a special lamp always use light energy and are called light-curing products.

- All other nail enhancement products use heat and are called heat-curing products.

- All polymers shrink when they form.

- Nail enhancement polymers shrink between 3-20%.

- Shrinkage greater than 12% can cause lifting, tip cracking, and other types of service breakdown.

- Chemical reactions that release small amounts of heat are called exothermic reactions.

- Exotherms can cause damage to the tissue and weaken the enhancement.

- The warmer the monomer, the faster it will cure.

- Faster set means more heat in a shorter time, which creates uncomfortably warm exotherms.

- The primary reason for unhealthy nail beds is overfiling and overpriming.

- Large-grit files and high-speed drills can be very damaging to the nail plate and nail bed.

- Excessive amounts of nail primer can seep through to the sensitive nail bed.

- Sculpting on metal forms may cause an exotherm, but rarely will it cause burning.

- Nail polishes, topcoats, and base coats also form coatings, but they do not polymerize.

- Uncross-linked polymers can absorb color between the polymer chains and become stained.

- Improperly cleaning brushes can contaminate them.

- Never pour monomer back into the original container.

- Yellowing and brittleness is one effect of improper consistency.

- NEVER use one manufacturer's liquid with another manufacturer's powder.

- NEVER blend your own "custom" nail enhancement products.

- The sun or tanning bed can cause some products to quickly discolor and lose flexibility.
- Properly formulated products are highly resistant to yellowing and premature aging.
- TSF resin is used to improve adhesion and toughen the polish coating.
- Nitrocellulose produces very hard, shiny surfaces.
- Nitrocellulose does not stick to the nail plate and is brittle.
- TSF resin softens and toughens the nitrocellulose, while improving adhesion.
- Nitrocellulose strengthens TSF resin and makes it hard and shiny.
- Plasticizers increase flexibility and wear of the polymer base.
- Prolonged use of formaldehyde causes the nails to become split, dry, and brittle.
- There is little reason to believe that toluene in nail polish is harmful to breathe.
- Base coats and topcoats are formulated with many of the same ingredients as polish.
- Topcoats have high amounts of the nitrocellulose polymer with extra plasticizer.
- Blowing on the polish will lower adhesion and gloss.
- Applying the second coat of polish too quickly is a major reason for the "orange peel" effect.

Questions

Chapter 5

1. What are coatings? Name the two main types.

2. Every type of product used to create nail enhancements does so by a chemical reaction called _____.

3. What are monomers and polymers? Define each and explain the differences.

4. What is the difference between a simple polymer and a cross-linked polymer?

5. After the monomers react, and a hard polymer is created, are the chemical reactions finished? Explain your answer.

6. Where does the initiator molecule get its energy? (Hint: two sources.)

7. Why do polymers shrink when they are created?

8. What is an exotherm? How can you tell when it is happening?

9. Do nail polishes and topcoats polymerize on the nail? Explain.

10. Explain how to test a nail enhancement product to see if it yellows *without* actually applying it to a client.

S I X

Understanding
Nail Enhancements – Part I

No one can say for certain when and where the very first nail extension was applied. Some clever manicurist tried strengthening a client's nails with the products dentists used to make dentures. A lot has changed since those first enhancements were applied. Nail technicians now have many new services and products to offer clients. However, these services all revolve around the nail enhancement. In this chapter you will use the information learned in Chapter 3 to discover how nail enhancements work. To properly understand the information below, it is very important that you have read Chapter 5 before continuing.

Family Ties: The Acrylics

Nail technicians use many types of products to create artificial nail enhancements. Light-cure gels, liquid-and-powder systems, wraps, and no-light gels all seem totally different and unrelated. Nothing could be further from the truth. The monomers used to make each of these are very closely related. In fact, they all come from the same chemical family, the acrylics.

The first artificial nail enhancement products were called acrylic nails. As you might imagine, they weren't very good by today's standards. But neither were the first cars, computers, or airplanes. All new products need time to reach their full potential. Still, many associate the word "acrylic" with those outdated products. They don't realize that all artificial nail enhancements are acrylic in nature. You can see why it is important to avoid using slang terms. It just creates confusion. But, just because these products are based on the acrylic family doesn't mean they're all the same. You wouldn't say all Americans or all Australians are the same. There are hundreds of kinds of acrylics. Liquid-and-powder systems are based on one branch of this family – the **methacrylates.** Wraps, no-light gels, and instant nail adhesives are based on another related branch – the **cyanoacrylates.** Light-curing gel products use methacrylates, but they also use **acrylates.** Each category has advantages and disadvantages. There are no perfect product types. None are ideal in every way or in every situation. In the next two chapters we will explore how they differ. We will also look at advantages and disadvantages of each.

Two-part Systems

The original nail enhancement products were two-part systems. These systems are still the most widely used type of nail enhancement in the world. Many years of experience and research have evolved these products far beyond those used by the first nail technicians. These early systems are often called "Liquid-and-Powder." The "liquid" is really a complex mixture of monomers. The "powder" is a polymer which contains the initiator and other additives. When nail technicians first began using these products, there was little or no product education. Unfortunately, many incorrect terms came into common use. It is very confusing to call monomers "the liquid" and polymers "the powder." Nail technicians will never gain their proper place in the professional beauty industry or in the eyes of their clients until they stop using such overly simplistic names.

These "liquids" are the *most sophisticated and high-tech products used in the entire beauty industry!* These same chemicals are used in lifesaving medical devices, computers, commercial jets, and on the space shuttle. What would you think of a NASA scientist who said, "Now, let's cover this thingamajig with some liquid and powder"? It is a terrible injustice to call them liquids. Nor does it give your clients much reason to believe that you are a true professional, using highly advanced systems and techniques. Throughout the rest of this book, these systems will be referred to by their proper names, monomers and polymers. Hopefully, nail technicians everywhere will do the same and do it with pride!

The Polymer Carrier

You learned in Chapter 5 that monomers join to create polymers. So, it might seem strange to mix liquid monomers and powdered polymers to create another polymer.

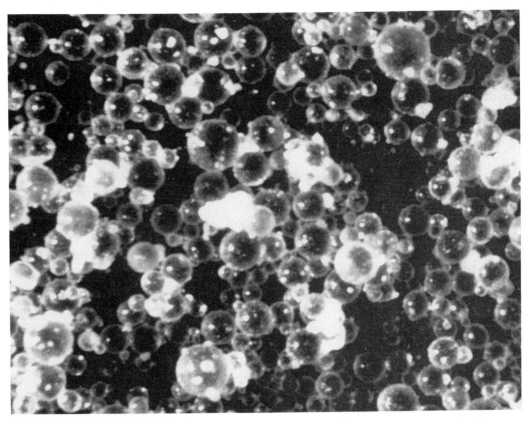

Fig. 6.1
Highly magnified beads of white tip powder. The large white chunks are titanium
dioxide, a whitening pigment. Smaller particles give some beads a frosted appearance.
(Courtesy Creative Nail Design Systems, Inc.)

This is exactly the case. Let's look at the powdered polymer first and understand its
role in the creation of a nail enhancement.

The polymer powder has an important role. It acts as a **carrier,** holding other ingredients. Several ingredients needed to make nail enhancements are coated on the outside of the polymer. A mineral called **titanium dioxide** is used to create a more natural appearance. This is the same pigment used in white housepaint. A tiny amount,
blended into the polymer, creates a natural coloration on the nail plate. Figure 6.1
shows a highly magnified bead of polymer powder coated with titanium dioxide.
Higher percentages are used to make white-tip polymers. White-tip polymers are
used to create extensions beyond the free edge and to give a "French manicure." An

extra-white tip polymer contains additional titanium dioxide. Of course, clear polymer powders use no titanium dioxide. This mineral is used because of its fantastic ability to whiten. Nothing does a better job. Strangely, the fine powder is extremely white, but a large crystal of titanium dioxide is clear and more brilliant than a diamond. Unfortunately, it is too soft and easily broken.

Dyes are sometimes added to give the polymer a pinkish or bluish color. These colors give a very pleasing appearance to the nail bed. Pink dyes will also cover-up yellowing and product discoloration. Blue coloration acts as an **optical brightener.** An optical brightener makes colors look brighter. Whites look whiter when a small amount of blue is added.

The polymer also carries a heat-sensitive initiator. In the last chapter, you discovered that an initiator was needed to energize the monomers. Monomer-and-polymer systems are heat curing. This is because the initiator is sensitive to heat. The initiator is usually **benzoyl peroxide,** the same ingredient used in acne creams. The heat of the room and hand is enough to break a molecule of benzoyl peroxide in half. Each half is capable of exciting or energizing a monomer. When a molecule breaks in half, it is called a free radical.

Free Radicals

Free radicals are very excited molecules that cause many kinds of chemical reactions. They can be found almost everywhere. For instance, hydrogen peroxide free radicals lift and deposit hair color. Our bodies use free radicals to perform thousands of vital functions each day. Free radicals also play a role in wrinkling and aging of skin. Many skin care products contain chemicals which eliminate free radicals. So you see, some free radicals are useful, others are not. The free radicals found on skin are very different from those used in nail enhancement products. Also, don't confuse benzoyl peroxide with the peroxide used for treating hair, hydrogen peroxide, which is much more aggressive than initiators used in nail enhancement products. That hasn't kept some marketers from suggesting that their "peroxide-free" products are better for the nail. This is silly and untrue. The benzoyl peroxide has NO damaging side effects on the nail plate.

A Radical Reaction

Free radicals are very important to nail enhancements, but don't worry that they will injure nail plates. Once a free radical excites the monomer, it is completely eliminated. Let's use what was learned in Chapter 5 to get a better picture of how these products work.

1. Monomer is mixed with a polymer containing benzoyl peroxide (initiator).

2. Heat breaks the initiator in half. This makes two free radicals.

3. Each free radical energizes a monomer. (Recall from Chapter 5, monomers don't like to be excited or energized.)

4. The energized monomers attach to another monomer's tail.

5. After attaching, they give the extra energy to the other monomer.

6. The second monomer doesn't want the energy either, so it attaches to the tail of another monomer and passes the energy again.

This cycle repeats itself billions of times making very long polymer chains. Each chain may contain millions of monomers. Notice that the polymer powder isn't mentioned. That's because it is only a carrier. The polymer powder does NOT chemically react. It carries the initiator to the monomer. Only the monomer can make a new polymer. The polymer powder does strengthen enhancement, as explained below. But, it does not become part of the new polymer chain. These growing chains wrap around the polymer and completely encase each particle.

Polymer Additives

The polymer powder contains other additives, as well. Sometimes, color stabilizers are added to prevent yellowing. Sunlight is one major cause of yellowing. It contains very high amounts of UV light which discolors enhancements and causes brittleness. **UV absorbers** are additives which prevent this damage. They absorb damaging UV light and change it into blue light or heat. In a sense, UV absorbers are like sunscreens for enhancements. They work on the same principle.

Calcium is sometimes added to polymers, but its benefits are questionable. Calcium certainly does *not* strengthen the nail plate. It cannot stimulate nail growth. In fact, it provides no benefit at all for the nail plate. Some believe that a small amount gives the product a slightly creamier consistency. However, in high concentrations it weakens the enhancement and causes premature service breakdown.

Making Polymer Powder

As you might suspect, the polymer powders start out as monomers. The process is very much like making a nail enhancement, except on a larger scale. Monomer is placed in a large mixer which may hold over 1000 gallons. Solvent is then added to dilute the monomer. The initiator and catalyst are added and the blend is mixed rapidly. After several hours, the monomer polymerizes into tiny beads. The solvent is drained away and the beads are then dried and packaged.

The bead sizes vary greatly. The size of very small things, like polymer powder particles, are measured in **microns.** Microns are easy to understand. A human hair is about 100 microns wide. A 50-micron particle is half as thick as a hair. Most polymer powder particles are around 50-100 microns. However, they can be as large as 125 microns or as small as ten microns ($^1/_{10}$ of a hair's thickness). The polymer powder particles shown in Figure 6.2 are highly magnified. You can see that they are not all the same size. It would be impossible to make them exactly the same size.

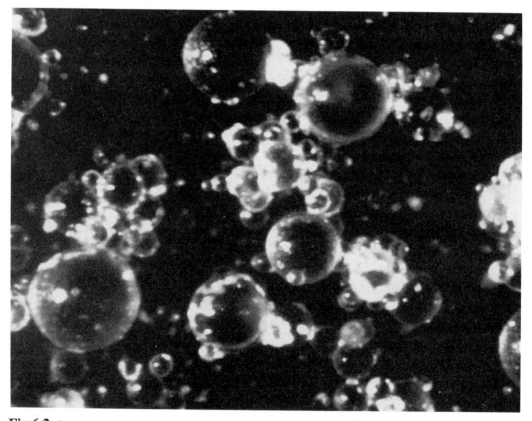

Fig.6.2
Highly magnified polymer powder particles. A wide range in particle size can be found in all polymer powders. *(Courtesy Creative Nail Design Systems, Inc.)*

A common misconception is that these powders are made by grinding. Grinding would be very expensive and unnecessary. It would also produce an inferior polymer powder. Manufacturers easily control the particle's size when the polymers are made. In other words, when the polymer is dried, it is already the correct size. Another misconception is that the polymer powders are sifted many times. This is untrue and also unnecessary. The polymer is passed through a screen to remove large chunks. However, additional sifting is unnecessary, costly and would not make the product any better – just more expensive.

Major Categories of Artificial Nail Enhancement Products

Cyanoacylates	Methacrylates	Acrylates
Wraps	Monomer and Polymer (Odorless and Odor-based)	UV Light Gels
No-light Gels	UV Light Gels	
Tip Adhesives		

Table 6.1
Three branches of the acrylic family and the products made from each category.

Composition

As shown in Table 6.1, both monomers and polymers are based on methacrylates. Methacrylates are a type of monomer. There are many kinds of methacrylates, but only a few are useful for artificial nail polymers. These different types are usually so similar that they can be thought of as sisters. Still, even sisters are different in many ways. The same is true for monomers. Powders are usually made from two "sister" monomers. These sisters are called methyl methacrylate and ethyl methacrylate. Methyl methacrylate monomer was used for many years to make artificial nails. It is no longer used because it caused too many allergic reactions. However, a polymer made from methyl methacrylate does not cause allergic reactions. Its sister, ethyl methacrylate, is the most widely used monomer in the nail industry. It is used to make odor-based monomer liquids. Polymer powder can be made either of ethyl or methyl methacrylate.

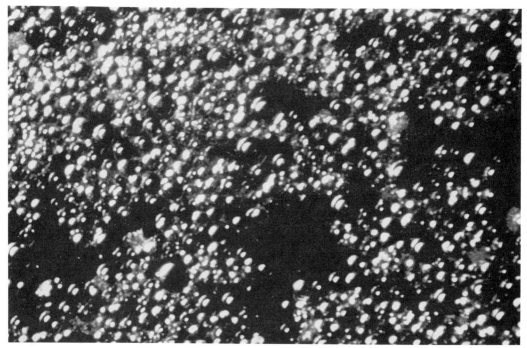

Fig. 6.3a
Incorrect ratio of monomer-to-polymer creates voids where no polymer can be found. The monomer-rich areas are black spaces in the highly magnified view. Fig. 6.3a depicts too wet of a consistency. *(Courtesy Creative Nail Design Systems, Inc.)*

Homopolymer versus Copolymer

A polymer made of only ethyl or only methyl is called a **homopolymer.** Homo means "same." In other words, the polymer was made entirely from the same monomer. To simplify things the ethyl polymer is called PEMA (the *E* is for ethyl). The methyl polymer is called PMMA (the first M is for methyl). Both PEMA and PMMA are homopolymers. Usually, a blend of both monomers is used to make polymer. In other words, the polymer chains contain both monomers, instead of just one. A polymer made from two or more monomers is called a **copolymer. Co** means "two or more working together."

Homopolymers made from ethyl monomer are more flexible. Homopolymers made from methyl monomer are harder and stronger. In general, copolymers blend the best of both monomers. Recall from Chapter 2 that toughness is a combination of

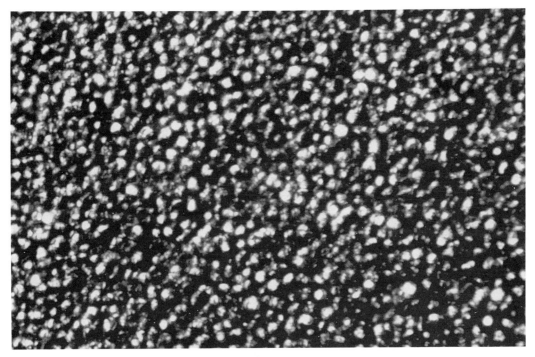

Fig. 6.3b
Correct consistency.

strength and flexibility. So, you can see why copolymers are tougher. Using two or more monomers allows manufacturers to create designer polymer blends. A polymer is made harder by using more methyl or flexibilized by adding more ethyl. Clearly, copolymers offer many advantages over homopolymers.

Strength Through Consistency Control

Consistency is determined by the amount of polymer powder used. If the proper consistency is used (see following page) the nail enhancement will contain the correct amount of polymer powder. For odor-based products, the enhancement will contain between 33-40% polymer. The polymer powder has dramatic effects on the artificial enhancement's performance. In fact, it gives the enhancement much of its strength. Figures 6.3a-b show a magnified view of monomer and polymer at both correct and incorrect ratios. When the monomer polymerizes, it surrounds each tiny bead. The polymer beads reinforce the entire enhancement. Too little polymer powder means less reinforcement and lower strength.

Nail technicians sometimes use extra monomer to smooth the surface of the enhancement. They don't realize that this lowers the consistency and reduces strength. This means excessive breakage. The highest strength is obtained by using the correct ratio of monomer-to-polymer. It is important to avoid using too wet a consistency. Table 6.2 is from actual laboratory data showing the strength of enhancements at different consistencies. As you can see, too much monomer or too much polymer can lower the enhancement's strength. Achieving the correct ratio takes a little practice, but the rewards are great. Clients will be happier and you will spend less time doing repairs. How this is done will be discussed in the next section.

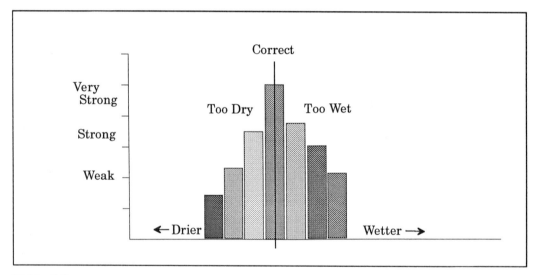

Table 6.2
Strength of artificial nail enhancements at various ratios of monomer and polymer.
(Courtesy Creative Nail Design Systems, Inc.)

Monomer Blends

The monomer is the most important part of the nail enhancement. Without monomer we would be limited to polish, base coats, and topcoats. Like polymer powder, these monomers come from the methacrylate family. Usually, odor-based products are mostly ethyl methacrylate. However, other monomers and additives are also used. Ethyl methacrylate only makes long, straight, polymer chains. By itself, it cannot form cross-links. (Remember, monomers normally join together in a head-to-tail fashion). Special monomers called cross-linkers must be added to obtain the three-dimensional net-like structures.

Besides cross-linkers, many other additives are used in monomer blends. For instance, UV absorbers are also put into the monomer liquid. Monomer blends can be simple mixtures containing only a few ingredients. Some are complex blends with ten or more ingredients. A common myth is that all products are alike. This is completely false. Some companies are not true manufacturers and sell products under their own private label. Even these products are different. The true manufacturer often custom blends a formula at the request of the seller. Some manufacturers of less expensive products want you to believe their products are the same as the expensive ones, but it just isn't so. A good rule to remember is…. "you get what you pay for." As you would imagine, economy products use basic formulas with the minimum amount of special ingredients. Special additives increase performance, but also increase cost. UV absorbers that reduce yellowing are one example. Flow modifiers and wetting agents are another. A **flow modifier** is an ingredient which reduces brush strokes on the surface. Brush marks seem to melt away or "self-level." They also improve workability. Wetting agents were discussed in detail in Chapter 4. These additives improve adhesion to the natural nail plate.

Catalysts

Catalysts are very important. By itself the initiator molecule is much too slow. A catalyst speeds things up. Without the catalyst, it would take days for the enhancement to harden. Remember, the initiator is the starting gun, but the catalyst is the trigger. Catalyst is usually only about 1% of the monomer, but it makes all the difference. You might think that adding more catalyst makes the chemical reaction go even faster. Strangely, the opposite happens. Adding more will make the enhancements set up slower. It will also make the artificial enhancement weaker and causes yellow discoloration. The extra catalyst makes the reaction happen too fast. Too many polymer chains start to grow. The result is an enhancement with many short polymer chains, and very few long chains. This gives the surface a "softer set." The enhancement becomes too flexible. When enhancements are too flexible, they bend and break more easily. So you can see, more flexible isn't always better. Some flexibility is important, but too much causes problems.

Inhibitors

Inhibitors are ingredients which prevent monomers from joining. In other words, inhibitors prevent polymerizations. Inhibitors are added to the monomer blend to improve shelf-life. Inhibitors prevent the monomer from turning to a thick, jelly-like substance. This is called **gelling.** Monomer will slowly turn to polymer if an inhibitor is not added. Without inhibitor, the product would gel within a few months. Inhibitor prevents gelling for up to 1 1/2 years, if properly stored. Improper storage deactivates inhibitor and causes gelling to happen very quickly. Excessive heat is the most common reason for product gelling in the bottle. Products should NEVER be stored in a warm place. Keep them away from windows. Store them in cool, dry locations. Keep products away from sources of heat, open flames, or sparks. Never put any product in the trunk of your car, especially in the summer. Even if there is no obvious gelling, your enhancements will be weaker and more prone to lifting.

Another common reason for product gelling is contamination. Once the monomer is poured out of the container, NEVER pour it back! Contaminants destroy the inhibitor. Unused monomer can be stored in a separate container and used to clean your brush. It *cannot* be reused, and *must* be disposed of properly.

Oxygen Inhibits, Too!

Many types of monomers are affected by oxygen. They cannot make polymers if too much oxygen is around. Oxygen affects the surface of the nail enhancement. It allows only a few monomers to join, resulting in a sticky, gooey layer that rolls off when filed. Deeper molecules are shielded from oxygen by the monomers near the surface. They are free to polymerize normally. This is often seen in odorless monomer-and-polymer systems, as well as in light-curing products.

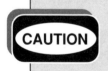

CAUTION This gooey layer is wet with monomers. You must avoid prolonged or repeated skin contact. Many technicians develop skin sensitivities from letting their arm or wrist rest in the filings.

Consistency Control

Consistency is the ratio of monomer-to-polymer. Extra monomer makes a consistency wetter. A drier consistency is made by using more polymer. Improper consistency is the number one reason nail technicians fail when using these products. The correct ratio of monomer-to-polymer must be used. Too dry a consistency causes breakage and lifting, but too wet a consistency is worse. If you go too wet, the enhancements may seem strong, flexible, and adhere well to the nail plate, *but don't be fooled.* All is not well! Too wet a consistency is one of the leading causes of allergic reaction in clients and nail technicians.

Wet Consistency	2 parts monomer to 1 part polymer
Medium-Wet Consistency	1 $\frac{1}{2}$ parts monomer to 1 part polymer
Dry Consistency	1 part monomer to 1 part polymer

Wet consistency will give better adhesion, but lower strength. This is because it contains less polymer. Too wet can mean big trouble. Besides causing allergic reactions, it can lead to cracking, lifting, and peeling. Dry consistencies have equal amounts of monomer and polymer. These offer the best strength, but less adhesion. Medium-wet consistencies give the best of both worlds. Medium-wet enhancements are strong and flexible, but they also have good adhesion.

There is an easy way to determine the proper consistency for most monomer-and-polymer products.

1. With a clean brush, make a bead in your normal fashion.

2. Carefully lay the bead on top of a clean, unfiled tip. Place the bead directly on the center or apex.

3. Do not pat or push down on the bead. It should form a small mound or dome.

4. Watch the bead for 15 seconds and note what you see.

Which of the following best describes your observations?

A. Does the bead begin to settle and flow out almost immediately? Does the height of the bead drop halfway or more in 15 seconds? Does the bead seem to lose most of its original shape? If you look carefully, can you see a ring of monomer around the base of the bead?

If you answered yes to *any* of these questions, your bead is probably too wet. If you answered yes to *all* of these questions, your ratio is probably greater than three parts liquid to one part powder.

WARNING

You are using the product incorrectly. You may experience tiny stress fractures and slight lifting near cuticles. You have also increased the chance that you and/or your clients will develop allergic reactions.

B. Does the bead melt out fairly slowly during the 15 seconds? After melting out, does it hold its shape? Does the overall height of the bead drop a little? Does the top of the mound fall by about one-fourth of the original height?

If you answer yes to *all* of the questions you are probably using a medium wet mixture. Good for you! Make sure you always stick to this procedure. You will be much less likely to have problems.

C. Does the bead hold its original shape and/or melt out very little? Does the bead's height and shape remain the same or almost the same? Does the bead seem to look lumpy or frosty?

A yes to *any* of these questions may mean you are using a dry consistency. Only odorless products require this ratio for strength and to lessen chances of allergic reactions. However, this is too dry for odor-based products. This mixture can lead to massive lifting of the product, sometimes in sheets. It can also cause brittle cracks.

Vital Importance

Nail technicians are often fooled into using too wet a consistency. Using wetter consistencies is the lazy way to make the surface smooth, but it causes far more problems than it solves. Smooth surfaces can be achieved with proper application at correct ratios. A high-quality product performs best at medium-wet ratios.

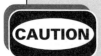

CAUTION

- NEVER go back and smooth the surface with more monomer.
- NEVER use pure monomer to "clean" around the edges, under the nail, or sidewalls.
- NEVER touch any monomer to the skin (including gels and wraps)!

Many serious problems can be related to the above. Don't fall into these traps. These bad habits are ghosts from the early years of the nail industry when there was no proper education. Don't be a victim of past mistakes and myths. More information on allergy and other skin ailments will be discussed in Chapter 9.

Other Additives

Many special additives are used to improve product performance. Plasticizers are an important example. **Plasticizers** improve flexibility and toughness. How? Empty air pockets exist between the millions of tangled polymer chains in a nail enhancement. These pockets are far too small to see, even with a microscope. These spaces can be detected only with very sensitive and specialized scientific equipment. If you could shrink down to the size of a molecule, the enhancement would look like a jungle of polymer vines. Between the vines would be many small spaces. Even though they are small, they are important. Plasticizers will fill these spaces. Just like motor oil lubricates your car engine, plasticizers can lubricate the polymer chains. They allow chains to slide and shift when they are hit or stressed. This tiny extra movement lets the polymer chains absorb shocks and impacts without breaking. They prevent cracking and make polymers tougher and more flexible.

Porcelain

Porcelain is incorrectly used to describe a monomer-and-polymer system. There have never been "porcelain" nails and never will be. Porcelain is made from a blend of special ceramic powders that are mixed with water then heated slowly to over 1500°F. Sound like any nail enhancement process you've ever seen?

Use Some Solvent Sense!

CAUTION: Never warm a solvent with an open flame, stove, blow dryer, or other similar devices. Solvents should be warmed with great care! Most are highly flammable. To warm the solvent, place the amount needed in a bottle just large enough to held all of the solvent. Warm only enough solvent to do the job. Loosen the cap of the "warming bottle" to allow vapors to escape. Place the warming bottle under a stream of hot running tap water, or in a bowl filled with hot tap water. Neither the water nor the solvent should be hotter than a steaming Jacuzzi® (110°F maximum). Take care to avoid any open flames, sparks, or other sources of ignition, *(i.e.,* cigarettes). Warm solvents and their vapors are even more flammable! For *more* information on sensible solvent safety, see Chapter 8.

Of course not! This is one of many old-fashioned ideas passed down from the days when our industry had no real education or information. Sadly, some still use this word to describe or market their products.

Removers

Cross-linking makes enhancements more resistant to solvents in nail polish and polish removers. Unfortunately, it also makes product removal more difficult. Only uncross-linked polymers dissolve in solvents. Cross-links prevent the enhancement from dissolving. Then how is the product removed? The solvent swells the polymer network until it breaks into chunks. The same effect is seen when a roll of paper towels is put into a bucket of water. The water doesn't dissolve the paper, but the roll will eventually break into pieces. It will break up even faster if you poke it with a stick. The enhancement will also swell more quickly if the solvent is slightly warm (see sidebar on previous page for more information). Warming the solvent can cut product removal time in half.

The most commonly used solvent for removal of nail products is acetone. Acetone is used for two reasons:

1. It is extremely efficient.
2. It is the safest solvent nail technicians can use, except for water.

Nonacetone removers can't compare for safety. Some are slightly faster, but they are more damaging to skin and are not as safe to breathe. More will be said about acetone and nonacetone products in later chapters.

Avoiding Allergic Reactions

Allergic reactions occur in every facet of the professional salon industry. Nail, skin, and hair services all can cause problems for the sensitive client. Fortunately, the vast majority of fingernail-related problems can be easily avoided – if you understand how! Allergic reactions are caused by prolonged or repeated contact. Therefore, skin problems do not occur "overnight." Acrylic liquids, wraps, and UV-light gels are good examples. In general, it takes from four to six months of repeated exposure for a client to become sensitive to these products.

Nail technicians are also at risk. Prolonged, repeated, or long-term exposures can cause anyone to become sensitive. This is what is called overexposure. Simply touching monomers doesn't cause sensitivities. It requires months of improper handling. Nail technicians sensitivities are often seen between the thumb and index finger. Why? Many nail technicians' constantly smooth brushes with their fingers. Eventually the area becomes sore and inflamed. Touching clients' skin with any monomer has the same effect. With each service the risk of sensitization increases. **Sensitization** is greatly increased or exaggerated sensitivity to products. It is extremely important that you always leave a $^1/_8''$ margin between the product and the skin.

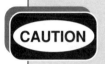
Never intentionally touch any nail enhancement product to the skin.

Methyl Methacrylate (MMA)

In the early 1970s nail technicians used monomer and polymer obtained from local dentists or medical supply stores. Many technicians became severely allergic to these dental products, because they didn't avoid skin contact. The culprit was the monomer, methyl methacrylate. Once it was determined that methyl methacrylate, also called MMA, caused intense allergic reactions, the FDA confiscated certain MMA-containing nail products and warned against its future use. The problem with MMA is that its small size allows it to penetrate the skin. This, in combination with several other factors, made it unsafe for use in our industry. Responsible manufacturers immediately changed to the much safer ethyl methacrylate. Ethyl methacrylate, also call EMA, is hundreds of times less likely to cause allergic reactions. However, skin contact should always be avoided with ALL artificial nail enhancement products. There are no exceptions to this rule!

The FDA's action was designed to protect the consumer, as well as, the nail technician. Methyl methacrylate not only caused serious skin reactions, it badly injured clients' nails. How? The monomer made nail enhancements that were extremely hard and rigid. Hard jams to the enhancement usually tore the nail plate or pulled it from the nail bed.

Long-term use of MMA can also cause respiratory problems in nail technicians. EMA is much safer and doesn't damage nail plates. But MMA is not gone. Unscrupulous, greedy individuals continue to sell MMA, despite the FDA warning. They know that nail technicians don't understand the dangers of using this monomer. They think they are just getting "harder nails." They don't realize they are jeopardizing their health and that of their clients. Nearly pure MMA monomer is usually sold to unsuspecting nail technicians. However, some of these unprincipled marketers blend small amounts into their professional products. If you suspect that you are being sold MMA or that another nail technician is using this monomer, call your State Board immediately. Let them investigate the matter.

Here are some of the warning signs of MMA.

1. Is the enhancement almost impossible to remove with a solvent?

These signs apply only to monomer-and-polymer systems. Some of these are true of UV light-cure gels, but they DO NOT contain MMA.

2. Does the product seem to set much harder and feel less flexible than other monomer-and-polymer systems?

3. Is it much more difficult to file? Only files with very coarse grits work?

4. Does the product smell different or stronger than other products?

These are the four warning signs of MMA. Anyone selling MMA is a danger to *all* nail technicians. Any nail technician who knowingly uses MMA is endangering their clients' and their own health. If you know of a nail technician who buys these dangerous products, you'd be doing yourself and the industry a favor if you reported your suspicions. Avoiding allergic reactions is the responsibility of everyone in the nail industry. Those who take this responsibility lightly are a risk to us all.

Mixing Powders

A common reason for sensitivity in clients is mixing product lines. Monomers work best with correct polymer. Never use one brand of polymer powder with another brand of monomer! The polymer powder must contain the right amount of initiator for that monomer. If the correct consistencies are used the enhancement does not cause skin sensitivities. Upset the delicate balance and this is no longer true. The wrong powders may not contain enough initiator. The balance can also be upset if the monomer contains too much catalyst for the polymer powder. The result? Extra monomer remains trapped inside the enhancement. Eventually, the extra monomer soaks through the nail plate and into the nail bed. This prolonged and repeated exposure is one of the leading causes of skin reactions. Unfortunately, several products are being marketed as "monomers for any powder." It is impossible to manufacture a monomer blend that would work with *any* polymer and with *any* percentage of initiator. The same is true for polymer powder. None works with *all* monomers!

Allergies can occur if the consistency is too wet. Consistencies that are too wet contain too little powder and initiator. Therefore, all the monomer doesn't react. Again, this extra monomer can soak through into the nail bed. Of course, overly wet mixtures easily run into the client's skin, further increasing the risk of sensitivity. Using extra large or oversize brushes usually make beads that are far too wet. The belly of a large brush can carry enough monomer for *four* medium-wet beads! In short, brushes that are too large don't save time – they can lead to allergic reactions.

Allergic reactions are easily avoided. Never use a brush that is too large for the job. Always use the correct powder with your monomer. Also remember, never touch the skin with monomer of any type, including wraps, adhesives, and UV gels. Wear gloves to prevent contact when pouring or transferring liquid and wash your hands often. All of these things will help protect healthy skin. You will learn more about allergies, why they occur, and how to avoid in coming chapters.

Damaged Nails?

A common myth among consumers is that nail enhancement products "damage" or "eat" the nail. This is completely untrue! You can verify this for yourself. Take a small clipping of natural nail plate and place it in a tightly capped bottle filled with monomer. You can keep this bottle at your station and show it to anyone who believes that the monomers eat or damage the nail plate. The nail will remain whole and unchanged. In 50 years when you retire and sell your chain of nail salons, before you take that trip around the world, look at that piece of nail plate. You'll be able to take it out of the bottle and see that it is the same – unchanged! You can do the same experiment with primer or any other nail enhancement product.

Nail products do not damage nails – *nail technicians damage nails!* Improper application procedures and improper product removal account for over 99% of the damage done in nail salons. It usually boils down to lack of knowledge, understanding, and awareness. Nail plate and cuticle damage is easy to avoid, but not by blaming the products. If your client's nail plates or cuticles are in bad shape, you are to blame. It is your job to keep the *entire* nail unit healthy. Accept that responsibility and you will be a success. Turn your head the other way or place the blame elsewhere and you will be a bad nail technician who deserves to fail. In fact, all the "good" nail technicians, clients, and manufacturers will be hoping you fail quickly!

You are a part of a billion-dollar professional industry. There is no room for nail technicians who have no regard for their own or their client's health. The information presented in this book will make you better educated than the "best" nail technicians of the last 25 years. You have access to information they never dreamed existed. Use this knowledge. Be the best you can be. You'll find it is easier in the long run and far more rewarding.

■ FAST TRACK

- The monomers used to make all enhancements come from the same chemical family, the acrylics.

- Monomer-and-polymer systems are based on one branch, called the methacrylates.

- Wraps, no-light gels, and instant nail adhesives are called cyanoacrylates.

- Light-curing gel products use methacrylates, but they also use acrylates.

- The polymer powder is the carrier for several key ingredients.

- The polymer carries a white mineral called titanium dioxide.

- Dyes are sometimes added to give the polymer a pinkish or bluish color.

- Blue coloration acts as an optical brightener. It makes colors look brighter.

- The polymer carries a heat sensitive initiator called benzoyl peroxide.

- Heat breaks benzoyl peroxide molecules in half, making two free radicals.

- Free radicals are excited molecules that cause many kinds of chemical reactions.

- Benzoyl peroxide has NO damaging side effects on the nail plate.

- Monomer is mixed with a polymer containing benzoyl peroxide (initiator).

- Heat causes the initiator to break in half and make two free radicals.

- Each free radical energizes a monomer.

- Energized monomers attach to the tail of another monomer, passing along the extra energy.

- The second monomer attaches to the tail of another monomer and passes the energy again.

- The polymer powder does NOT chemically react.

- Only monomer can make new polymer.

- These growing chains wrap around the polymer powder, completely encasing it.

- UV absorbers prevent discoloration caused by absorbing damaging UV light.

- Calcium doesn't strengthen the nail plate or stimulate nail growth.

- Polymer powder bead sizes are measured in microns.

- A human hair is about 100 microns wide.

- Most polymer powder particles are around 50-100 microns.

- Polymer powders are not made by grinding.

- Polymer powder can be made either of ethyl or methyl methacrylate.

- Polymer made of only one type of monomer is called a homopolymer.

- A polymer made from two or more monomers is called a copolymer.

- Copolymers give better toughness.

- Consistency is determined by the amount of polymer powder used.

- The polymer powder gives the enhancement much of its strength.

- Too little polymer powder means less reinforcement and lower strength.

- Excessive amounts of monomer lowers the consistency and reduces strength.

- The highest strength is obtained when using the correct ratio of monomer to polymer.

- It is important to avoid using too wet a consistency.

- Inhibitors are ingredients which prevent polymerizations.

- Inhibitors are added to the monomer blend to improve shelf life and prevent gelling.

- Never keep any product in the trunk of your car, especially in the summer.

- NEVER pour monomer back into the bottle.

- Oxygen inhibition results in a sticky, gooey layer that rolls off when filed.

- Technicians can develop skin sensitivities from letting their arm or wrist lie in filings.

- Consistency is the ratio of monomer-to-polymer.

- Improper consistency is the number one reason nail technicians fail when using these products.

- Too dry a consistency causes breakage and lifting.

- Too wet a consistency is one of the leading causes of allergic reaction.

- Wet consistency gives better adhesion, but lower strength.

- Medium wet enhancements are strong, flexible, and have good adhesion.

- NEVER go back and smooth the surface with more monomer.

- NEVER use pure monomer to "clean" around the edges, under the nail, or sidewalls.

- NEVER touch any monomer to the skin (including gels and wraps)!

- Plastizers improve flexibility and toughness.

- Cross-linking makes enhancements more resistant to solvents.

- Cross-linking also makes product removal more difficult.

- Acetone is a commonly used solvent because it is extremely efficient and very safe.

- Methyl methacrylate causes intense allergic reactions and should never be used.

- Allergic reactions can be easily avoided – if you understand how!

- Allergic reactions are caused by prolonged or repeated contact.

- In general, allergies develop after four to six months of repeated exposure.

- Sensitization is greatly increased or exaggerated sensitivity to products.

- Never intentionally touch any nail enhancement product to the skin.

- Monomers should only be used with the polymer they are sold with.

- It is impossible to make monomer blends that work with all polymer powders.

- Allergies can occur if the consistency is too wet.

- Overly wet mixtures run into the client's skin, increasing the risk of sensitivity.

- Extra large or oversize brushes usually make bead consistencies which are too wet.

- Brushes that are too large don't save time – they can lead to allergic reactions.

- Nail products do not damage nails – nail technicians damage nails!

- Improper application and improper removal account for over 99% of damaged nails.

Questions

Chapter 6

1. What is the name of the chemical family of all enhancement monomer coatings and adhesives?

2. What is a UV absorber and how does it work?

3. How big are most polymer powder particles?

4. What does excessive amounts of monomer do to the strength of the nail enhancement?

5. What are inhibitors? Why are they used?

6. _____ of a consistency, _____ brushes, and using the _____ powder with a monomer are some of the leading causes of allergic reaction.

7. If you performed the bead test for checking your consistency, as described in the chapter, describe what a medium-wet bead would look like.

8. Why is it unsafe to use methyl methacrylate-containing products?

9. Explain how to safely warm solvents designed for removing enhancements.

10. What should you do if you suspect that someone is selling methyl methacrylate?

SEVEN

Understanding Nail Enhancements – Part II

Wraps are another popular technique for creating artificial nail enhancements. Wraps can be used to coat the nail plate or add strength to thin, weak nails. Advanced techniques also allow technicians to create extensions beyond the free edge. Even though it is difficult to build up or reshape the nail plate with a wrap, they are simple to use and can be quite beautiful.

You will use the information learned in Chapter 5 to discover how enhancements work. To properly understand this chapter it is very important that you have read Chapter 5 before continuing.

Wraps System

The Monomer

The monomers used to create wraps are called cyanoacrylates. As shown in Table 6.1 (Chapter 6), they too are members of the acrylic family. These are the same monomers used to create many fast setting adhesives such as Krazy Glue.® However, professional nail products are specifically designed for use on fingernails. They are far superior for this application. These monomers polymerize in a very unique way. The monomers are sensitive to alcohol, water, and weak alkaline (bases) substances. In large amounts they cause almost-instant polymerization. A drop of water or alcohol on wrap monomers will cause **"shock curing."** They will harden quickly and turn cloudy white. They turn cloudy because shock curing causes thousands of microscopic cracks. You can't see them with your eye, but the cracks scatter light reflecting from the surface. This gives the polymer a cloudy appearance. Of course, small amounts of these substances cause slower, controlled reactions. This results in polymers which are clear, flexible, and strong. Although they have many advantages, wraps have the disadvantage of not being cross-linked. As you know, cross-linking builds strong, three dimensional networks that resist staining. Uncross-linked polymers are easily attacked by polish and polish remover solvents. Cross-linking also allows durable extensions to be built beyond the free edge. Since cyanoacrylate monomers are not cross-linked, they are best used for natural nail and tip overlays.

Water-sensitive monomers must be protected from moisture in the air. These monomers are sold in containers with small nozzles. This prevents air moisture from gelling or thickening the product. As with other monomers, inhibitors are used to prevent gelling. Even so, leaving a container open for too long will thicken the product fairly quickly. You may think moisture sensitivity is a negative. Actually, it is a big positive. The nail plate contains enough moisture to polymerize wrap monomers. Just touching the nail plate is often enough to react the monomers. Some products are designed to work in this way. These can be brush-on monomers or may be applied with a nozzle. These products use nail plate moisture to harden and need no additional catalyst.

Catalysts

Catalysts speed up the polymerization and reduce cure time from minutes to seconds. Spray or brush-on catalyst causes an almost-instantaneous reaction. The catalysts are usually weak alkaline substances (the label may list them as "aromatic amines"). As you learned in the last chapter, rapid reactions can cause rapid heat build-up. Incorrectly used, these catalysts may heat the nail plate to a blistering 170°F. A small amount of warming is beneficial and will improve enhancement strength. However, pain-causing heat may cause serious burns to nail beds. This excessive heat may damage sensitive tissue and weaken the enhancement.

To avoid overheating, some catalyst must be sprayed from a distance. This is a potential source of overexposure if no precautions are used. The same ingredients used as wrap catalyst are found in many artificial nail enhancement products. If used properly, the ingredient is safe. However, careless and uncontrolled spraying may create problems. As with most chemicals used in the professional salon, it is important to avoid excessive skin contact. Fortunately, overexposure only happens with prolonged and repeated contact. Overexposure is easy to avoid by using a common sense approach. For example, technicians should wear dust masks designed for mists and sprays to avoid excessive inhalation. Ventilation systems which vent vapors to the outdoors are also required. Residual catalyst will coat the tabletop and should be cleaned up regularly. Long-term skin contact with this residue could lead to overexposure. In short, wear the proper mask while spraying. Always use proper ventilation, and regular housekeeping is a must. More information on masks and other tips for working safely will be discussed in Chapter 8.

Tip Adhesives

Certain types of cyanoacrylates are used as tip adhesives. These products are formulated differently. They are also sensitive to moisture. However, these adhesives are designed to work best when there is no air. Most set slowly or turn to a rubbery gel in the presence of air. Oxygen inhibits the cure. When the air supply is cut off, the adhesive sets quickly. This feature is a great benefit for nail technicians. It allows maximum working time and a quick set once the tip is properly placed. In general, thinner adhesives set faster, but this is not always good. Usually, extremely fast setting adhesives give lower-strength bonds. If you have a client whose tips just don't seem to hold or if they separate after a few weeks, try a slower-setting, thicker adhesive.

Thin adhesives will only hold if there are no small gaps between the tip and nail plate. If the nail plate doesn't closely match the tip, a thicker adhesive will work better. For example, ski-jump or spoon-shaped nail plates are ideal for thicker adhesives. Thicker adhesives fill gaps that thinner products cannot. Still, don't use too much. These adhesives work best if only a small amount is used – just enough to do the job. Thickened adhesives usually contain dissolved methacrylate polymer. It is similar to the powder used in the two-part monomer-and-polymer systems. It gives the bond more strength, especially in gaps. Since these adhesives are not crosslinked, they are affected by moisture. Clients who frequently wet their hands should be warned that all cyanoacrylates are moisture sensitive. This is true of both adhesives and wraps. Instruct them to wear gloves whenever possible.

Glues

The word "glue" is commonly misused. People often use it to mean anything sticky. However, glues are really a name for a certain type of adhesive. True glues are adhesives made from animal protein, hide, bones, and hooves. No professional nail adhesive is made from animal by-products, so it is incorrect to call them glues. The proper term is *adhesive.* In the professional nail industry we use advanced monomer adhesives, not glue!

Other Additives

Special additives separate professional products from those found in supermarkets. General-purpose products work well around the home, but they can't compete with professional products. Adhesives and wrap monomers are mixed with special additives designed to improve adhesion, strength, and flexibility. Some also contain special wetting agents which help improve nail adhesion, strength, and clarity.

Wrap Fabrics

Various types of fabrics are used to reinforce the polymer wrap coating. These fabrics provide support and added strength to the coating. There are three fabrics in wide use: fiberglass, silk, and linen. The type of fabric used is generally not as important as the weave. The weave and the thickness of the fabric determine its usefulness. A very loosely woven fabric would not reinforce as much as one with a closer weave. However, tightly woven fabrics create other problems. The monomer must be able to penetrate the weave. Monomer must soak completely through the fabric. Otherwise, it sets on top of the fabric. This causes small spaces or voids between the monomer and the fabric's fibers. These spaces scatter light, making the enhancement look cloudy. The voids also create weak areas where cracks may later develop and grow.

If the monomer absorbs easily into the fabric, the coating will be stronger and clearer. This is called wetting and was discussed in Chapter 4. If you recall, proper wetting allows the monomer to cover the surface more thoroughly, penetrate deeper, and hold tighter. Proper wetting depends upon the fabric and product composition. Special wetting agents called **silanes** are additives which allow faster penetration of the fibers. These are coated on the outside of most fabrics.

Fiberglass and silk are very similar in properties. Generally, silk is more easily wetted. Better wetting usually creates a more natural appearance. However, if properly applied, both silk and fiberglass create thin, strong, and natural-looking nail enhancements. Linens tend to be thicker and tightly woven. It is difficult for the monomer to penetrate most linens. The result is thick, cloudy coatings that must be worn with nail polish to cover the unnatural appearance. Because the monomer can't completely wet the linen, these fabrics can lift and peel away (called delamination; See Chapter 4). Some feel that since linen is a stronger fabric it must give strong nail enhancements, but this is untrue. Medium-weave silk, and fiberglass provide the best overall combination of strength, retention, clarity, and wetting.

Some fabrics are coated with an adhesive backing. The backing helps hold the fabric in place. If the adhesive is applied too thickly, it can interfere with proper adhesion

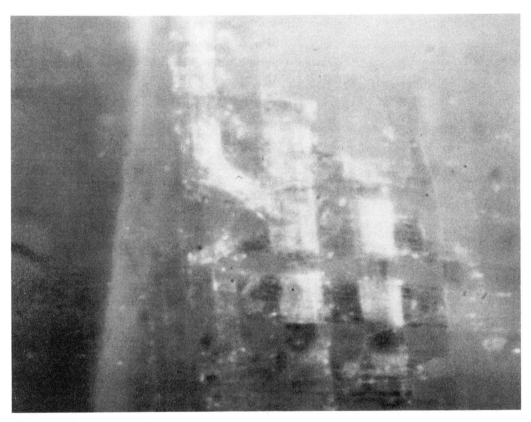

Fig. 7.1
Highly magnified section of an improperly wetted fiberglass fabric used for a wrap enhancement. *(Courtesy Creative Nail Design Systems, Inc.)*

by reducing fabric wetting. Skin oil and other contaminants can also block wetting. Touching fabric will deposit large amounts of skin oil on the fabric. This can lead to peeling, lifting, and cracking. Oil makes the fabric more noticeable on the nail plate. Figure 7.1 shows the effect of improperly wetted fabric. Avoid touching fabric excessively, especially with dirty hands. This helps eliminate many problems, including lifting.

Removal

One of the best features of wraps is their easy removal. As you know, uncross-linked polymers quickly break down in solvents. Acetone is especially safe and efficient for wrap removal. As you would expect, warming the solvent can cut product removal time in half. (See sidebar on page 83 for information on safely warming solvents.) However, undiluted acetone is not a good choice for polish removal. Most

Don't Do It!

Sometimes, nail technicians will sprinkle polymer powder over wrap monomer and adhesives. This is a foolish practice. It may appear to work, but over time, the initiator in the polymer powder weakens the bond. It will also make wraps less durable and can cause discoloration. Always follow manufacturer's instructions: If they don't instruct you to sprinkle powder on the monomer, don't do it. Ignoring manufacturer's instructions can cause unforeseeable problems and potential legal trouble for you. If a client has any problems, you could be found guilty of negligence, simply because you ignored the instructions!

solvents will attack the surface of the wrap. The result is tiny microscopic cracks which lead to breakage. Some polish removers are diluted for polish removal. A diluted solvent will cause less damage to wraps.

Wrap Safety

All professional nail chemicals can be used safely. Wraps are no exception. However, improper use can cause a variety of problems. For instance, excessive catalyst may burn and damage nail beds. Care must be used when spraying any substance. Overexposure to vapors and mist are more likely to occur while spraying. As with all professional nail enhancement products, wrap products MUST be used with appropriate ventilation. Proper ventilation is one of the most important things you can do to improve safety in the salon. Mist masks should also be worn when spraying wrap catalyst. These special masks look like ordinary dust masks, but are designed to prevent overexposure to mist and sprays. Breathing excessive amounts of vapors can cause shortness of breath and difficulty breathing. Unless you have asthma or other lung disorders, this is usually a result of long-term overexposure. Be smart and don't take chances. Protect yourself before you develop problems. Mist masks and proper ventilation can help prevent overexposure. For more information on mist masks and which ventilation systems work best in the salon see Chapter 10.

Avoid Skin Contact

Wrap and adhesive monomers react quickly with moisture, so great care must be taken to avoid skin contact. Skin is bonded together almost instantly by these substances. A large droplet can release enough heat to damage the skin. Should this happen, don't panic! Cool the area as quickly as possible with cold tap water. If the fingers become bonded, soak them in acetone until the bond is dissolved. NEVER attempt to "pry" the skin apart. This will rip and tear the skin, only worsening the problem. The same is true of clothing or other items. If anything becomes bonded to the skin, soak with acetone until the bond completely dissolves. Never open or use the product over your lap or near your face. Wearing gloves while using these substances will greatly reduce the chance of accidents. Remember, prolonged or repeated contact can lead to allergic reaction and permanent skin sensitivity.

Eye Protection

Many accidents with wrap and adhesive monomers involve the eyes. Usually, these occur while removing stuck caps or pin closures. ALWAYS point the tip away from you or your client when opening the container. Also, ALWAYS wear safety eye protection when using wraps.

WARNING Accidents may happen if you carry wrap monomers or adhesives in your purse. The container is sometimes mistaken for eyedrops or nasal spray and *can be accidentally poured into the eyes or squirted into the nose.*

Children sometimes are injured if these substances are left in their reach. Serious damage can occur if these substances get in the eye. If this ever happens, quickly cool the eye with lots of cold running water to prevent burns. After rinsing, the monomer will be hardened. DO NOT rub or touch the eye area. A doctor can very easily open the stuck eyelid, usually without any damage to the eye or loss of eyesight. It is important to avoid touching, rubbing, or pulling. This is what causes the most damage and may lead to permanent loss of eyesight.

UV Gel Systems

UV or visible light-curing gels have been around for many years, but have recently regained popularity. The first generation of gels had lots of problems. However, the second generation has overcome many of these challenges with advanced scientific technology. Newer products are beginning to meet the tough demands of the professional nail industry. As you learned in Chapter 5, gel systems can use either visible light or UV light to create nail enhancements. For simplicity, we will use the term "gel" when referring to both types of products.

No-Light Gel

The term "no-light gel" is misleading. The name suggests that these are like regular UV gels, but they need no light. Not true! These products are wrap monomers that have been thickened to have a gel-like appearance. They should be used and handled as any other wrap product. They have most of the benefit and disadvantages of other wrap products. Many feel that the gel wrap product is easier to use because it is thicker. However, thicker monomers will not wet fabric as easily.

Monomer versus Oligomer

These products are very similar to two-part, monomer-and-polymer systems. In some instances, gels share many of the same ingredients. Gels are often sold as being "not acrylics." This is false! They most certainly *are* from the acrylic family. As you recall from Chapter 5, gel monomers are based on both the methacrylates and the acrylates families.

Why are gels so different? Polymerizing monomers with UV or visible light is not very efficient. It is difficult to get UV light deep into the gel. If gels were made entirely of monomers, most of the gel would not turn into polymer. One way to improve efficiency is to prejoin some of the monomers into short chains. These short chains are neither monomers nor polymers. They are in between. These short chains are called **oligomers.** Oligomers make it easier to create polymers. An oligomer is a single chain that is several thousand monomers long. Joining a few hundred oligomers is much faster and easier than joining a million individual monomers. Why are gels so thick? Nail enhancement monomers are liquids and polymers are solids. So, it makes sense that oligomers are in between. This is why gels are "gel-like" in consistency. Now you can understand one of the disadvantages of most gel systems. They are more difficult to use because of the heavy consistency and their tendency to be stringy. On the positive side, the thicker consistency reduces evaporation and odor.

New technology will soon change all of this. As gel ingredients become more sophisticated, gel products will improve. Someday, many of the problems associated with gels will no longer haunt nail technicians. Gels certainly have a bright future in the professional nail industry.

Initiator and Light

As discussed in Chapter 5, some initiators use heat energy and others use light. It is easy to keep light away from gels so the initiator, catalyst, and oligomers can be combined together into a single product. This is possibly one of gels' greatest advantages. They come premixed and ready to use. Still, no system is perfect. Each has advantages and disadvantages. Curing with UV or visible light is more convenient, but raises special problems that must be addressed.

Initiators are activated by light. The light must penetrate completely through the gel to polymerize all of the oligomers. Unfortunately, this doesn't occur. Thick coatings of gel allow less light to reach the bottom layers. In Europe where gels are used extensively, they attempt to overcome this with powerful UV lights. These European systems use 38-45 watts of UV light. American systems tend to be far lower, usually eight watts. UV bulbs emit only UV-A, so there is little danger (see sidebar, "Don't Watch That UV-A Exposure," Chapter 5, page 54). However, the high-wattage lamps are far more expensive. Higher wattages can cause problems, too. Remember, when polymers cure too quickly, they release large amounts of heat in a short period. This can cause serious and damaging burns to the nail bed. You can see now why getting a complete cure is very difficult (Figures 7.2a-b).

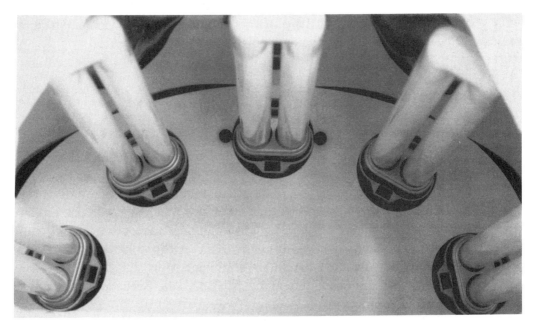

Fig. 7.2a
Close-up of a five-bulb, 45-watt German gel lamp. *(Courtesy Paul Rollins.)*

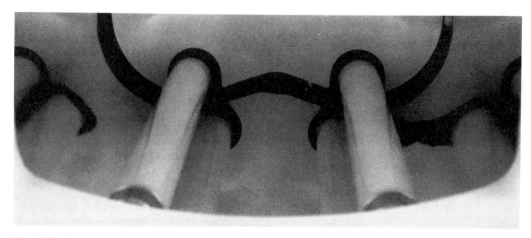

Fig. 7.2a
Close-up of a two-bulb, 8-watt American gel lamp. *(Courtesy Paul Rollins.)*

Skin Sensitivity and Proper Cure

Incomplete cure is a huge problem in the nail industry. As you learned in Chapter 6, using the wrong polymer with a monomer or using too wet a consistency leads to incomplete cure. Monomer residues may cause allergic reactions. The same occurs with gel systems. A large percentage of the enhancement may contain uncured oligomer. Several factors determine the degree or percentage of cure:

- Thickness of gel layer

- Length of cure

- Bulb condition

- Type of oligomer

The thickness of the gel coating has a great effect on the degree of cure. As a rule, the thicker the coating, the less efficient the cure. It is much better to use three or four thin coats rather than one or two thick coats. Thinner coats allow more light to penetrate the layer. Also, the hands will be under the gel light longer if more coatings are used. Another advantage is reduced shrinkage. Gels shrink more than any other type of enhancement. Using thinner coats reduces the effects of shrinkage, as will be described later in this chapter.

The time that gels spend under the light is extremely important! The longer the enhancements remain in the UV light, the more completely they cure. Some manufacturers don't recommend longer exposures. They worry that nail technicians will see this as an inconvenience. Also, some products yellow more with long light exposure. Still, longer cure times are better. More UV light means less uncured oligomer and stronger nail enhancements. Remember, just because the enhancement is hard does not mean that it is fully cured. Always use a timer to ensure the correct light exposure. Never shorten the recommended time. If you use multiple thin coatings, you won't need to increase the time. Of course, this depends on the UV bulbs and their condition.

Bulb condition is vital to the success of gel enhancements. UV gel lamps become ineffective many months before they burn out. After about six months of normal use a bulb has less than half its original UV energy. UV bulbs should be changed twice per year even if they look fine. If the product seems to set slower than normal, change the bulbs immediately. It is a good idea to keep a spare set of bulbs around. Dirty bulbs also lower UV strength. Clean the bulbs whenever needed. At least once per week is recommended. If the bulbs become too dirty to clean, discard them and replace them with new bulbs. Skimping on bulbs will cost far more in the long run. Improperly cured gels are prone to service breakdown and will increase the chance of allergic reactions for both you and your clients.

Finally, the type of oligomer used plays an important role in skin allergy. As mentioned above, both methacrylates and acrylates are used as oligomers in gels. Methacrylates are far less likely to cause allergic reactions, but they polymerize slowly. Many formulations use acrylates to speed up curing. Although acrylates cure much faster, they are more likely to cause allergic reactions. For this reason, acrylate monomers are rarely used in monomer-and-polymer formulations. The stickiness of gels also contributes to allergies. Sticky gels are more likely to remain on implements and skin. Gels should NEVER be allowed to touch the skin. NEVER touch your client's cuticles, either. If contact occurs, immediately cleanse the area with soap and water. Keep brush handles, files, containers, and implements free of gel.

Skin contact with all gel nail enhancement products must be carefully avoided. Gels are the *most likely* nail enhancement product to cause allergies. Does this mean they are unsafe and should not be used? Of course not! Any nail enhancement product can cause allergies if used incorrectly. It is your professional responsibility to see that they don't! This is done by ensuring correct use. If you follow manufacturer's instructions and use the information presented in this book, you can avoid these problems.

Oxygen prevents surface curing. Gel formulations often show the same effect. Some oligomers can't join together if oxygen is present. The result? A sticky, gooey surface layer that must be removed with a solvent or file.

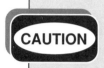 This gooey layer is rich in uncured oligomers! You must avoid prolonged or repeated skin contact. Many technicians develop skin sensitivities from letting their arm or wrist lie in the filings or by exposing their fingers when wiping with a solvent.

Shrinkage

In Chapter 5 you learned that all polymers shrink when they are cured. Wraps shrink between 5-9% and, monomer-and-polymer systems shrink between 6-10%. Gel enhancement products shrink up to 20%! Shrinkage is normal, but above 12% causes many problems. Lifting, tip cracking, and other types of service breakdown are often caused by excessive shrinkage.

Clients can sometimes feel the effects of excessive shrinkage. They may comment that the enhancement feels tight on the nail bed. Other symptoms are throbbing or warmth below the nail plate. This may lead to tender, sore fingertips. The symptoms may occur immediately or up to 24 hours later. This depends on how much the gel shrinks. After a few days, the discomfort diminishes, but might not entirely disappear. Excessive shrinkage is not only discomforting, it can cause damage or trauma to the nail bed. For example, the nail plate may separate from the bed. Usually it begins as a small white area at the free edge or hyponychium. Excessive shrinkage squeezes the nail plate causing it to pop free from the track that holds it against the bed (see Figure 1.4). Once the separation starts it easily travels further under the nail plate. In Chapter 1 you learned that the hyponychium forms a watertight seal. This seal prevents bacteria, fungi, and viruses from attacking the nail bed. Separations allow infections to take hold under the nail plate. Nail technicians are often surprised when clients develop infections. The client is blamed, but it is usually the nail technician's fault. Any trauma to the nail plate can lead to infection. Other causes of trauma are overfiling, heavy abrasives and drills, overpriming and wearing enhancements that are too long.

Nail technicians can minimize shrinkage by using multiple, thinner coats of gel – the best way to keep the nail plate thick and healthy! Thin, weak nails are easily damaged by excessive shrinkage and other kinds of trauma. The nail plate is the foundation for the enhancement. Remember, clients pay you to care for their fingernails FIRST, *then* to give them beautiful nails. Keep the natural nail plate and surrounding tissue healthy and they are less likely to have problems.

Exothermic Reactions

In Chapter 5 you learned that monomers release a small amount of heat when they join. This is called an exothermic reaction. Products that release heat very quickly will feel warmer. Rapid heat buildup can occur with certain gel formulations. This is generally caused by a poor choice of ingredients in the product. Excessive heat can also be a sign that there is an imbalance between the catalyst and initiator.

Damaged nail beds are extra sensitive to this heat. The primary reason for damaged nail beds is overfiling or "roughing up" the nail plate. The heat created from rough abrasives and heavy-handed filing drills are usually the cause. Gel products which use primer (methacrylic acid) in formulation can also make nail bed tissue more sensitive.

Removal of Gels

Most gels are difficult to remove. This is because they are highly cross-linked and resistant to many solvents. Usually, the product must be filed from the nail plate. This can damage the plate and underlying bed if not performed with care. One way to minimize the problem is to apply thinner coatings. The heavy consistency often causes gel users to apply the product too thickly. This creates unnatural and unsightly enhancements and makes removal very difficult.

Gel enhancements should only be removed when it is absolutely necessary. A common myth is that enhancements should be taken off every few months to let the nail plate "breathe." There is no scientific evidence to support this notion. Nail plates do not require time to breathe, nor are they *capable* of breathing. Each time product is removed and reapplied, the underlying nail plate becomes thinner and weaker. This is especially true when the gel is picked or pried from the nail plate. Improper removal is a crime against the client's nails. It is a major reason for natural nail damage. Nail enhancements should NEVER be picked, nipped, or pried from the nail plate. These are not gentle techniques. Each will rip up layers of natural nail plate. Proper removal of gels is a time-consuming process. You must take your time or the client's nails will suffer the consequences. If the nails must be removed use the following guidelines:

1. Slowly file (not drill) the enhancement with a medium-grit file, leaving a very thin layer of product. Do not file all the way to the natural nail plate.

2. Soak in warm product remover (see "Use Some Solvent Sense!," Chapter 6, page 88).

3. Once softened, scrape the remaining product away with a wooden pusher stick.

"Better-for-the-Nail" Claims

Some believe that gel enhancement products are "better" for the natural nail. This is absolutely false! In fact, gels are such a challenge to remove that improper or repeated removal causes great damage to the natural nail plate. Remember, *no one type of nail enhancement product is better for the nail plate than another!* What is truly "better for the nail"? That is easy to answer. The best thing for the natural nail are highly skilled, educated, and conscientious nail professionals. They are the natural nail's best friend. Good nail technicians protect and nurture the nail plate. Don't be fooled. Professional nail enhancement products don't damage the natural nail. Nail technicians are generally responsible for almost all of their client's nail damage and disease. Any product can be applied and removed safely. It is up to YOU to use your knowledge and skill to see that it happens.

The Future of Gels

Gels are constantly improving. This will continue as the science and technology behind them advances. Gels have the potential to become widely used and valuable tools, but this cannot happen until nail technicians also improve. Many useful ingredients cannot be used in gel formulation because too many nail technicians are careless and sloppy. Proper application and removal and avoiding skin contact are the key issues. Once all nail professionals begin to use their tools in an appropriate and professional manner, only then will enhancement products reach their true potential. If products are to improve and advance, nail technicians must do the same!

■ FAST TRACK

- ■ The monomers used to create wraps are called cyanoacrylates.

- ■ Cyanoacrylates are sensitive to alcohol, water, and weak alkaline (bases) substances.

- Large amounts of catalyst cause almost instant polymerization or shock curing.

- Shock curing causes thousands of microscopic cracks which cloud the surface.

- Slower polymerizations make polymers clear, flexible, and strong.

- Wraps have the disadvantage of not being cross-linked.

- Uncross-linked polymers are easily attacked by polish and polish remover solvents.

- Cyanoacrylates are water sensitive and must be protected from moisture in the air.

- The nail plate contains enough moisture to polymerize wrap monomers.

- Catalysts reduce cure time from minutes to seconds.

- Incorrectly used, these catalysts may heat the nail plate to a blistering 170°F.

- Technicians should wear mist masks designed for sprays to avoid excessive inhalation.

- Long-term skin contact with catalyst residue could lead to overexposure.

- Certain types of cyanoacrylates are used as tip adhesives.

- Extremely fast setting adhesives give lower-strength bonds.

- Thin adhesives work best when there are no gaps between the tip and nail plate.

- Thickened adhesives give the bond more strength, especially in gaps.

- Adhesives are not cross-linked; they are affected by moisture and solvents.

- True glues are adhesives made from animal protein, hide, bones, and hooves.

- The wrap fabrics in widest use are fiberglass, silk, and linen.

- Weave and the thickness of the fabric determine its usefulness.

- The monomer must penetrate the weave or the enhancement will be weak and cloudy.

- Proper wetting depends upon the fabric, product composition, and wetting agents.

- Generally, silk is more easily wetted and gives a more natural appearance.

- Linens tend to be thicker and tightly woven.

- Medium-weave silk and fiberglass provide the best overall combination of strength, retention, clarity, and wetting.

- Skin oil and other contaminants block wetting and lead to peeling, lifting, and cracking.

- Acetone is especially safe and efficient for product removal.

- Diluted solvents cause less damage to wraps.

- Skin is bonded together almost instantly by wrap monomers.

- NEVER attempt to "pry" bonded skin apart.

- Never open or use the product over your lap or near your face.

- Prolonged or repeated contact can lead to allergic reaction.

- Always point the tip away from you or your client when opening the container.

- Always wear safety eye protection when using wraps.

- No-light gels are thickened wrap monomers with a gel-like appearance.

- Gel monomers are based on both the methacrylates and the acrylates families.

- It is difficult to get UV light deep into a gel coating.

- Efficiency is improved if some monomers are prejoined into short chains called oligomers.

- Light must penetrate completely through the gel to polymerize all of the oligomers.

- A large percentage of the enhancement may contain uncured oligomer.

- Factors which determine cure efficiency are: thickness of gel layer, length of cure, UV bulb condition, and type of oligomer.

- Thinner coats allow more light to penetrate the layer.

- Gels shrink more than any other type of enhancement.

- Thinner coats reduce the effects of shrinkage.

- More UV light means less uncured oligomer and stronger nail enhancements.

- A UV bulb has less than half the UV energy after about six months of normal use.

- UV bulbs should be changed twice per year, even if they look fine.

- Dirty bulbs also lower UV strength.

- Methacrylates are far less likely to cause allergic reactions than acrylates.

- Gels should NEVER be allowed to touch the skin.

- NEVER touch your client's cuticles with gel.

- Keep brush handles, files, containers, and implements free of gel oligomers.

- Skin contact with all gel nail enhancement product must be carefully avoided.

- Used incorrectly, gel is the nail enhancement product most likely to cause allergies.

- Oxygen prevents surface curing in many gel formulations.

- Skin contact with the gooey surface layer must be avoided.

- Wraps shrink between 5-9%, monomer-and-polymer systems shrink between 6-10%.

- Gel enhancement products shrink up to 20%.

- Shrinkage above 12% may causes lifting, tip cracking, and other types of service breakdown.

- Excessive shrinkage can cause damage or trauma to the nail bed.

- Nail trauma can create a space under the plate allowing infections to take hold.

- Any trauma to the nail plate can lead to infection.

- Trauma is also caused by overfiling, heavy abrasives and drills, and overpriming.

- Thin, weak nails are easily damaged by excessive shrinkage and other trauma.

- Clients pay you to care for their fingernails FIRST, *then* to give them beautiful nails.

- Damaged nail beds are extra sensitive to heat.

- The primary cause of damage to nail beds is overfiling or "roughing up" the nail plate.

- Most gels are difficult to remove because they are highly cross-linked.

- There is no scientific evidence for the myth that enhancements must be removed to let the plate "breathe."

- Nail enhancements should NEVER be picked, nipped, or pried from the nail plate.

- Gel enhancement products are no safer or better for the natural nail than other systems.

- Improper or repeated removal of gels causes great damage to the natural nail plate.

- Good nail technicians protect and nurture the nail plate.

- Nail technicians are generally responsible for almost all their clients' nail damage and disease.

Questions

Chapter 7

1. What is the monomer used to create wraps?

2. Wrap monomers will polymerize when exposed to _____ , _____ , or _____ .

3. In general, extremely fast setting adhesives give _____ strength bonds.

4. The _____ and the _____ of the wrap fabric determine its usefulness.

5. Name three important pieces of safety equipment required for working with wrap products.

6. A(n) _____ is a short chain of monomers that is not long enough to be a polymer.

7. List the four factors which determine the degree or percentage of cure in gel systems.

8. Gels are the _____ nail enhancement product to cause allergies.
   a. most likely   b. least likely

9. What generally causes the nail plate to separate from the nail bed? Give four examples.

10. Which type of nail enhancement product is "best" or "safest" for the natural nail?

EIGHT

The Safe Salon

Every chemical used in the professional salon industry can be used safely. On the other hand, every chemical can be potentially dangerous. What makes a product safe or dangerous? You do! How you use your professional tools is the key. If you understand them, use them cautiously, correctly, and wisely, then neither you or your client will ever be injured. In this chapter you will learn the basics of working safely.

Chemophobia

What is a chemical? Most people believe chemicals are dangerous or toxic substances. Ask someone what they think about "chemicals." They might mention toxic waste dumps or factories dumping poisonous waste into streams. Actually, everything you can see or touch is a chemical, except for light and electricity. Air is a combination of many chemicals (*i.e.,* oxygen, hydrogen, and nitrogen). Clean, pure mountain stream water is a chemical. A new born baby's skin is 100% chemicals.

Why do people only think of chemicals in a negative way? It is because of the overdramatized and exaggerated images created by the media. These images are misleading and inaccurate. The truth is, 99% of the chemicals you will come in contact with in your life are completely safe and beneficial. Unfortunately, most reporters have no understanding of chemistry. The news almost always uses the word "chemical" in a scary, negative way. They have created a negative-information plague called **Chemophobia,** the fear of chemicals. Like most phobias, the fear isn't based on facts! What is the cure for Chemophobia? Knowledge and understanding! No one is afraid of the things they understand. We fear only what we don't understand. Knowing your chemical tools will put you in complete control. That's the good news. Working safely is very easy to do.

Water is the most common salon chemical. Water can be very dangerous! Water is such a dangerous chemical it can kill you in minutes. You don't believe it? Try sticking your head in a bucket of water for five minutes. Of course, no one would do such a foolish thing. But, why do we know better than do this? Since you were very young, your parents taught you about the potential hazards of water. We learn that it is dangerous to swim after a big meal or use a blow dryer in the bathtub. We were taught not to drive fast on wet pavement. We learned all the rules for using this potentially deadly chemical. The same is true for salon chemicals. There are rules that must be obeyed when working with all chemicals. If these rules are disobeyed, we may suffer the consequences. Always remember, every chemical can be safe and every chemical can also be dangerous – it is up to you!

Time Out

If you are serious about becoming a professional nail technician, you must take the time to learn the rules of working safely – why risk the consequences? Learn to use products correctly and SAFELY. Study the manufacturer's educational literature and warning labels. Always use products in strict accordance with the manufacturer's instructions and follow the rules of working safely. Remember: safety and health come first!

The Rules of Working Safely

Is it possible to work safely with potentially dangerous chemicals? Of course it is, but you must learn how. Safety doesn't just happen. You must learn the facts and obey the rules of working safely.

Fact #1: No chemical in the world can be harmful unless you OVEREXPOSE yourself.

The most important thing to know about chemicals is said in the "Overexposure Principle." This rule says, "Every chemical substance has a safe and unsafe level of exposure. Simply touching, inhaling, or smelling a potentially hazardous substance can't harm you. Exceeding the safe level of exposure is the danger you must learn to avoid."

Some chemicals are dangerous even in tiny amounts. They are not suited for salon use. Professional products are formulated to be as safe as possible. Still, no nail product or other cosmetic chemical is free from all risks. A normally safe product can become dangerous if used incorrectly. Even gardeners and mechanics must follow safe working procedures.

Rule #1: Look for ways to reduce your exposure.

If you follow this one rule, you will be safe in the salon. Everything you will learn in this chapter will teach you how to reduce your exposure. You will also find that Materiel Safety Data Sheets (MSDS) are another important source of safety information.

Material Safety Data Sheets

The MSDS provides information to all chemical workers, including nail technicians. MSDSs help firefighters deal with chemical fires or clean up large spills. This information often helps doctors treat accidental poisonings. The MSDS provides important information about each product you use. Any professional product that contains a potentially hazardous substance has an MSDS.

Here is a brief list of what you can learn from a MSDS:

- Potentially hazardous ingredients found in each product
- Proper storage and fire prevention
- Ways to prevent hazardous chemicals from entering your body
- The short- and long-term health effects of overexposure
- Early warning signs of product overexposure
- Emergency first aid advice
- Emergency phone numbers
- Safe handling techniques

Routes of Entry

There are only three ways that a potentially hazardous chemical can enter your body. These three ways are called the "**routes of entry.**" If you block these, then you will automatically lower your exposure. These routes are:

1. *Inhalation* by breathing vapors, mists, or dusts.

2. *Absorption* through the skin or broken tissue.

3. Unintentional or accidental *ingestion*.

The MSDS will advise you which route of entry is possible for a product. Lowering your exposure is easier if you know which products require special ventilation and which should be kept off the skin.

Health Effects

The MSDS explains both the short- and long-term effects of overexposure. Short-term or **acute** effects result from overexposure for usually less than six months. Short-term effects are "early warning signs" of overexposure. Some examples of acute effects are headaches, nausea, scratchy throat, coughing, or rashes. Acute effects such as these are rarely permanent and usually will quickly disappear when overexposure ends.

Long-term or **chronic** effects can also occur with overexposure or misuse. Some chronic effects occur after only six months, while others take many years of repeated overexposure. Remember, adverse health effects are not what *will* happen. Quite the contrary! These dangers *may* happen, if you MISUSE or abuse the product for long periods. The products you use are tools, not toys! Treat them with respect and you can avoid problems.

Signs and Symptoms of Overexposure

The human body is very rugged and complex. The body usually gives early warning signs of overexposure. Unfortunately, these signs and symptoms are often ignored. For instance, overexposure to some solvents can make you feel very tired or keep you from sleeping. Overexposure can cause headaches, nausea, angry or frustrated feelings, nosebleeds, coughs, dizziness, tingling fingers and toes, dry or scratchy nose and throat, puffy red and irritated skin, itching, and many other symptoms.

Watching for these acute symptoms will help you avoid more serious, long-term problems. Pay attention to what your body tells you. Remember, if you lower your exposure, acute symptoms usually go away. Why feel ill when it is easy to avoid?

Emergency and First Aid Treatment

If a serious accident happened in your salon, what would you do? Should you induce vomiting or give the victim something to drink? Use a hot compress or cold?

Elevate the feet or the head? Wash with running water? We find out how unprepared we are for accidents after it is too late.

Fact #2: Accidents usually occur when they are least expected.

The MSDS will answer your questions during a time of crisis. The MSDS provides specific instructions for accidental spills, splashes, or ingestion. Keep them handy; they will prove to be very useful.

The next rule is a familiar one.

Rule #2: Be Prepared! Plan ahead for accidents.

What would you do if a small child ran up to your table and drank your nail primer? Similar incidents happen many times each year! By the time you remember where you put the poison control center's phone number it could be too late. Plan ahead: you may save a life! The MSDS will provide emergency phone numbers. Also, it is wise to find out the number for the local poison control center and hospital emergency room. Post them by the phone…. just in case.

Safe Handling Techniques

Every profession requires different tools and techniques. Knowing how to handle these tools is very important. A carpenter wouldn't use a screwdriver to hammer a nail. The same is true for professional salon chemicals. Each chemical requires different handlings for safe use. For example, quickly evaporating monomer and solvents require appropriate ventilation. Otherwise, over time the vapors may cause overexposure. Safety glasses prevent liquids from splashing in the eyes. Other products may require a special type of glove or extra precautions to prevent fires. Manufacturer's instructions and the MSDS will both guide you. If either of these suggest that you wear safety glasses, it is for good reason.

There is lots of information on the MSDS. Become familiar with reading them. Properly using these important resources is the wisest move you can make. Nail technology is changing faster than any other facet of the beauty industry. Keeping pace means keeping up with these changes. Your education doesn't end when you leave school. It just begins!

Blocking the Routes of Entry

Working safely is surprisingly easy! Even so, each year many experienced nail technicians suffer needless harm or injury. The rules of safety are designed to protect you and prevent problems. Remember, chemicals can only enter your body in three ways. If you block these routes you will lower your exposure to safe levels.

Fact #3: All liquids evaporate and form vapors.

Just because you don't smell anything doesn't mean there are no vapors in the air. Volatile solvents are those which evaporate very quickly. Some liquids evaporate slowly, but they still create vapors. Monomers are also very volatile. What is the best, easiest, and least-expensive way to avoid excessive inhalation of vapors?

Rule #3: Keep products capped or covered when not in use. Also, regularly empty waste containers.

If vapors never escape into the air, you don't have to worry about being overexposed. Closing product containers will drastically reduce the amount of vapor in the air. Besides, it will also help keep your products fresh and effective. An open container is an accident that is waiting to happen. If you use volatile monomers, always use a dappen dish with a hole in the lid. A small marble over the hole will prevent evaporation. When monomers evaporate, they change in composition. This can lead to yellowing, lifting, and breakage. Quickly wipe up spilled monomer and other chemicals. Use a metal waste container with a pop-up lid. This will help keep vapors out of the air and reduce the chance of fire. Don't forget to empty the waste container often.

Fact #4: Mists are difficult to control and potentially hazardous to breathe.

Mists are actually tiny liquid droplets. These droplets will rapidly evaporate into the air. Spraying any chemical into the air increases the risk of overexposure. Pressurized aerosol containers produce very fine and lingering mists. A fine mist is difficult to control and usually more hazardous to inhale (*i.e.,* pressurized wrap catalyst). Pump sprayers create larger droplets, which are less hazardous. Besides, pumps are better for the environment than pressurized cans. Avoid spraying excessive amounts of product into the air. Use pump sprayers whenever possible.

Rule #4: Avoid pressurized spray cans and use metal waste containers with pop-up lids.

Surgical-type masks (often called dust masks) are completely *ineffective* against vapors. These masks should only be used to keep dust particles out of your lungs. Vapor molecules are so small that they pass easily through a dust mask. These masks provide ZERO protection against vapors. They don't even help a little!

Fact #5: A vapor molecule is many hundreds of times smaller than a dust particle.

Some high-quality masks are also effective against mists. These are called mist-rated masks. The instructions that come with the masks will tell you if they can be used for both dusts and mists. However, they too are completely ineffective against vapors.

Rule #5: Never use a dust mask to protect yourself from vapors. Vapors are far too small to be "filtered" by dust masks. Use a mist mask if you spray anything.

Dusts

It shouldn't be surprising that prolonged inhalation of excessive amounts of nail filings may be harmful. Not because nail filings are a particularly dangerous type of dust, but breathing large amounts of ANY dusts (even house dust) for long periods may be harmful.

Fact #6: Any type of dust can accumulate in the lungs and cause overexposure.

Our lungs can handle a lot of dusts. The body has many ways of removing and disposing of inhaled dusts. When you inhale more than the lungs can handle, however, you increase your risks. Wearing a dust mask can prevent this. You should always wear a dust mask when filing, *especially* if you use a drill. Drills make much smaller dust particles than files or emery boards. Smaller particles lodge deeper in the lungs. This makes them more hazardous to your health. Larger particles are less harmful. Just about any particle you can easily see is considered large. They usually fall on the tabletop and are easily removed. Small particles may float around for forty minutes or longer before coming to rest. Then the slightest breeze will send them back into your air. Nothing you can buy will do a better job of protecting your lungs than a simple dust mask. Also, throw away dust masks every few days. They're disposable and become ineffective if used too long.

Your client may wish to wear a dust mask, too. That's fine, if it makes them feel better. But, can your client be overexposed to nail dust? No way! Remember the Overexposure Principle? Inhaling dust isn't harmful. Exceeding the safe level of exposure for long periods increases the risk. Your clients run no risk of overexposure because they aren't there long enough. You are exposed to more salon chemicals every four days than they are in a year! Explain the Overexposure Principle to your clients. Tell them that you are only taking steps to protect yourself. They will understand and be more at ease. You will also find that they become more confident in your knowledge, skills, and abilities.

Rule #6: Always wear a dust mask when filing, especially if you use a drill.

Dangerous Misconceptions

What is the most dangerous misconception about chemicals in the salon industry? Many believe that they can tell how safe or dangerous a chemical is simply by its odor! WRONG! A chemical's smell has absolutely nothing to do with its safety. Some of the most dangerous substances known have very sweet, pleasant fragrances.

Fact #7: Odors themselves are not dangerous. In fact, odors can help you work safer.

Using products or ventilation systems that "cover up" or "remove odors" from the salon will not protect your health. Simply removing odors will not make the air safer to breathe. Odors are no indication of product safety. Odors are the nail technician's friend. Odors can warn against overexposure danger. An odor is nothing more than vapors touching the sensitive detectors in the nose. After the vapors leave the nose and enter the lungs, odor is no longer important. You are asking for trouble if you use odor to judge product safety.

Rule #7: Never judge product safety by odor.

Don't listen to fast-talking salespeople that claim their ventilation systems make the salon air "fresh smelling" or will "remove chemical odors." Most of these systems are inadequate. They cannot do a proper job when it comes to protecting you. In Chapter 10, you will learn more about proper ventilation.

Working Smart

Question: What does a coffee cup, a piece of chocolate, and a sack lunch have in common?

Give up? These are all ways that nail technicians EAT their chemical products. "Who would eat their chemicals?" you might ask. Sadly, nail technicians eat far more product than they realize.

- Coffee cups can easily collect dusts. Hot liquids, like coffee and tea, will also absorb vapors right out of the air.

- When someone offers you a piece of chocolate or you dodge into the kitchen for a cookie – how many people think to first wash their hands?

- A common salon practice is to keep sack lunches in the refrigerator where products are stored. While you are working, the food is busy absorbing a dose of chemical vapors. Bread is especially good at absorbing vapors.

Fact #8: Federal regulations prohibit eating in areas where potentially hazardous chemicals are used.

This means salons, too! Accidental product ingestion is very easy to do in the salon. If you need to eat in a hurry, never do it at your station. Besides being unsanitary and illegal, it is a foolish chance to take with your health.

Rule #8: Never eat or drink in the salon. Always store food away from salon chemicals and wash your hands before eating or going to the restroom.

Protect Your Eyes

Accidents involving the eyes are a serious danger in salons. Solvents in the eye can be very painful and may cause severe damage. Primer, wrap monomers and adhesives, or phenolic disinfectant solutions in the eyes are worse! Each of these can cause permanent eye injury or blindness. Imagine what it is like to be blind. It could happen if you are not careful to protect your vision.

Fact #9: Each time you unsafely mix, open a container, or apply nail enhancement products, you could lose your vision.

Wear eye protection whenever there is the slightest chance that a liquid product could get into your eyes. *Eye injuries account for approximately 45% of the cosmetic-related injuries seen in hospital emergency rooms.* Many of these are students and salon professionals.

Rule #9: You should wear approved safety glasses whenever you work and should give your client a pair, as well.

Your client may love you and think you are the greatest nail technician in the world. But, if you accidentally splash primer or wrap monomer in their eyes, you have lost a friend and gained a lawsuit! You are responsible for the client's safety while in your care. If you ignore that responsibility, you may regret it one day.

If you wear prescription glasses you are in luck. Have your local optometrist make you a pair of prescription safety glasses. It is 100% tax deductible and much better than a Seeing Eye® dog!

Fact #10: Soft contact lenses can absorb vapors from the air.

Wearing contacts in the salon is risky. Vapors will collect in soft contacts and make them unwearable. Even if you wear safety glasses, vapors are still absorbed. The contaminated lens can etch the surface of the eye and cause permanent damage. Should an accidental splash occur, the liquid will "wick" under the lens. This will make proper cleaning of the eye more difficult.

Rule #10: Never wear contact lenses in the salon and always wash your hands before touching the eye area.

Many of these rules are just simple common sense. When using salon chemicals, common sense can save you from pain and suffering. Learn these chemical safety rules and obey them!

Scare Your Clients?

What if your client sees you putting on safety glasses and a dust mask, or following any of the other rules of safety? Many worry that it might scare the client. No one ever lost business because they worked safely or showed concern for a customer's well-being. Can you imagine them leaving you and going down the street to the salon that doesn't do any of these things? Would you if you were in their shoes? Of course not! If anything, they will respect you and appreciate your work even more. They will realize that there is a lot more to "doing nails" than filing and buffing. You should really be worrying that your client will think you *don't* work safely. Then you may lose them to someone who does!

Proper Storage Conditions

Improper storage of your chemical products can create many problems. Improper storage may destroy the product or shorten the shelf life. It may also cause a fire or explosion. Freezing temperatures, excessive heat, or sunlight adversely affects many products.

Flammable products must be stored away from heat, sparks, or open flame (*i.e.,* away from cigarettes and window sills). NEVER carry any product in a car trunk. Many salon chemicals are more flammable than gasoline. The MSDS will also help you to avoid other dangerous conditions. For example, dangerous mixtures which may emit hazardous vapors or cause fires.

Toxicity

Toxic substances are usually considered dangerous poisons. The news media uses the term often and most people shudder when it is mentioned. Should nail technicians avoid products that are toxic? The answer to this question will surprise you.

Paracelus, a famous 14th-century physician, was the first to study and understand toxic substances. He said, *"All substances are poisons; there is none which is not a poison. Only the right dose differentiates a poison and a remedy."*

Over the last 500 years, the public has forgotten what Paracelus discovered. The Overexposure Principle is the modern day interpretation of what he learned. If you remember, this principle also says that the dose level (overexposure) determines toxicity. Paracelus is correct; *everything* is a poison; therefore, we must avoid EVERYTHING, including cuticle oils and skin creams. Of course, this is foolish. Obviously, something is wrong with the way we define toxicity. How do scientists define "toxic"? They use the following guideline to determine the true risks to humans:

Fact #11: A chemical is considered to be relatively nontoxic only if drinking a quart or more won't cause death.

Next time someone tells you a product is *nontoxic,* think about this definition. This type of claim is actually very silly and deceptive. Saltwater is very toxic to drink. Still, we can safely swim in the ocean without fear of poisoning. Rubbing alcohol is also very toxic, but we manage to use it quite easily.

Rule #11: Treat all chemical products with respect. Don't be fooled by marketing terms like "nontoxic, "natural," and "organic."

Organic simply means the chemical contains carbon in its structure. Most things on Earth are organic. Cow dung, poison ivy, and road tar are all 100% organic and natural. *Natural* simply means "occurs in nature." Nature is a wicked place. It is filled with poisonous substances. "Natural" doesn't mean a product is safe, wholesome, or even better.

Carcinogenesis

According to the news, nearly everything causes cancer, right?

Fact #12: There are many millions of chemicals. Of these millions, fewer than 500 are suspected to cause cancer in humans. Many of these known cancer-causing agents are only dangerous at extremely high doses and long-term exposures.

Cancer-causing chemicals are rare. The majority of cancers are caused by cigarettes and hepatitis. Don't let exaggerated news reports frighten you. If you work safely, it is extremely unlikely that your products will give you cancer. The cancer risks from cigarettes are hundreds (maybe thousands) of times greater than any salon product you use. Even chemicals which may cause serious illness usually do so only if you are overexposed for prolonged periods.

Rule #12: Don't judge a chemical by what it CAN do. What's important is how easily you can prevent the potential hazard.

Sometimes people hear what a chemical "can" do and become frightened. Remember, "can" is a lot different than "will." Alcohol (in beer and wine) "can" cause liver damage.... if you drink a couple of quarts a day for five years! It won't happen because you have a margarita with lunch. Overexposure to many salon chemicals can cause illness, but this is so easy to avoid. These substances can be used safely, without posing a health risk. That is what Paracelus has been trying to tell us for 500 years.

Rule #13: There is no need to fear chemicals. Instead, be careful and wise.

Ultimately, YOU are responsible for preventing accidents and protecting your health! Learn what you can about working safely and always obey the rules. You may become the best nail technician in the world, but it won't mean anything if you harm yourself in the process. Don't just *talk* about working safely, *it only works if you really do it!*

Cumulative Trauma Disorders

Cumulative trauma disorder (CTD) is also known as repetitive motion disorder. CTDs are the fastest-growing type of occupational-related injury. CTD is actually the name of several different conditions. Each can cause painful and crippling illness that may become permanent if not treated. **Carpel tunnel syndrome** is the most common CTD. This illness affects the hands and wrists of many nail technicians. The carpel tunnel is a small passage in a wrist bone. It houses a nerve which runs from the fingers into the arm. Repetitive motions can injure this area and create pressure on the nerve.

The injury is almost always caused by repetitive motions such as typing or filing nails. Constant vibration from tools can also cause or aggravate the condition. Although the nerve is pinched in the wrist, pain and numbness often spread into the arm and fingers. If ignored, CTDs usually become worse and are often disabling. Continued injury can permanently damage the nerve. Other things, besides repetitive motion and vibrations, can cause CTDs. Sitting or working in the same position, awkward reaching, stretching, or twisting may damage the carpel tunnel nerve.

Symptoms for CTDs are:

- Pain

- Numbness

- Aching

- Stiffness

- Tingling

- Weakness

- Swelling

If you experience any of these symptoms pay close attention to how you work. You can often determine which motions cause the pain. However, it can be difficult to solve the problem without proper advice. It would be wise to seek medical attention immediately before it is too late to correct the problem. This is why it is important to recognize these symptoms. Early attention can reverse CTDs.

What to Do?

There are many things nail technicians can do to avoid CTDs:

- Always sit in a natural, unstrained position.

- Change positions often.

- Take frequent stretch breaks, even if they are only for a few seconds.

- Avoid using tools that vibrate excessively.

- Wear gloves that fit well.

- Hold wrists straight and avoid bending them while filing or using a brush.

- Don't hunch over the client's nails.

- Stop work and stretch or shake out your hands periodically.

- Develop a regular routine for exercising and stretching arms, wrists, and hands.

An easy and effective exercise is to press your hand on a flat surface while stretching your fingers and wrist for five seconds. You can ease symptoms with ice and ibuprofen or aspirin. However, if you develop symptoms it is important to see a doctor. Your doctor will be able to objectively see your problem and make recommendations that you might not think about. Remember, it won't go away on its own. You must learn to avoid the injury and give the body a chance to heal. CTDs are easy to prevent and correct. Don't take chances with your hands. You'll need them!

Sanitation Information

Do you wonder which type of disinfectant works best? Are you interested in learning more about viruses, fungi, and bacteria and how they spread? Ever wonder if it is possible to transmit diseases in the salon? You can find the answers to all your questions in:

HIV/AIDS & Hepatitis

Everything You Need to Know to Protect Yourself and Others

by Douglas Schoon

Milady Publishing

1-800-998-7498

This useful and informative book is written for salon professionals, but provides important information for everyone concerned about preventing the spread of contagious disease. It makes a perfect companion to this book and is very interesting reading.

Where To Get Equipment

If you are wondering where to find safety equipment for the salon, contact Lab Safety Supply at 1-800-356-2501. This company sells equipment for every type of business, including salons. Ask for a free copy of their latest general catalog. It contains many useful items ranging from dust and mist masks to gloves and safety glasses. They also have a technical help line that can answer many of your safety-related questions.

■ FAST TRACK

- Every chemical used in the professional salon industry can be used safely.

- Everything you can see or touch is a chemical, except for light and electricity.

- Of the chemicals you will come in contact with in your life, 99% are safe and beneficial.

- No chemical in the world can be harmful unless you OVEREXPOSURE yourself.

- The Overexposure Principle says, "Every chemical substance has a safe and unsafe level of exposure. Simply touching, inhaling, or smelling a potentially hazardous substance can't harm you. Exceeding the safe level of exposure is the danger you must learn to avoid."

- Look for ways to reduce your exposure to safe levels.

- The Materiel Safety Data Sheets (MSDS) are an important source of information.

- Chemicals can only enter your body in three ways; called the "routes of entry."

- The MSDS explains both the short- and long-term effects of overexposure.

- Short-term effects are early warning signs of overexposure.

- Acute effects are rarely permanent.

- Accidents usually occur when they are least expected.

- Be prepared! Plan ahead for accidents.

- All liquids evaporate and form vapors.

- Monomers are another example of products which are very volatile.

- Keep products capped or covered when not in use.

- Regularly empty waste containers.

- Closing product containers will drastically reduce vapors in the air.

- Mists are difficult to control and potentially hazardous to breathe.

- Spraying any chemical into the air increases the risk of overexposure.

- Pressurized aerosol containers produce very fine and lingering mists.

- Pump sprayers create larger droplets which are less hazardous.

- Avoid pressurized spray cans and use metal waste containers with pop-up lids.

- Dust masks provide ZERO protection against vapors.

- A vapor molecule is many hundreds of times smaller than a dust particle.

- Never use a dust mask to protect yourself from vapors.

- Vapors are far too small to be "filtered" by dust masks.

- Use a mist mask if you spray anything.

- Any type of dust can accumulate in the lungs and cause overexposure.

- Drills make the smallest dust particles which lodge deeper in the lungs.

- Your clients run no risk of being overexposed to dusts or vapors in the salon.

- Always wear a dust mask when filing, especially if you use a drill.

- A chemical's smell has absolutely nothing to do with safety.

- Never eat or drink in the salon.

- Always store food away from salon chemicals and wash your hands before eating or going to the restroom.

- Each time you unsafely mix, open a container, or use enhancement products, you risk your vision.

- Soft contact lenses can absorb vapors from the air.

- Never wear contact lenses in the salon.

- Always wash your hands before touching the eye area.

- Improper storage may destroy a product or shorten the shelf life.

- Flammable products must be stored away from heat, sparks, or open flame.

- NEVER carry any product in a car trunk.

- Many salon chemicals are more flammable than gasoline.

- All substances are poisons; there is none which is not a poison. The right dose differentiates a poison and a remedy.

- A chemical is considered to be relatively nontoxic only if drinking a quart or more won't cause death.

- "Organic" simply means the chemical contains carbon in its structure.

- "Natural" means nothing more than "occurs in nature."

- Cancer-causing chemicals are rare.

- The cancer risks from cigarettes are hundreds (even thousands) of times greater than any salon product you use.

- There is no need to fear chemicals: Instead, be careful and wise.

- Cumulative trauma disorder (CTD) is also known as repetitive motion disorder.

- CTDs are the fastest growing type of occupational-related injury.

- Carpel tunnel syndrome is the most common CTD.

Questions

Chapter 8

1. What do the Overexposure Principle and Paracelus's philosophy have in common?

2. List five important pieces of information found on an MSDS.

3. Name the routes of entry and give examples of a safety technique that can block each route.

4. What is the cheapest and easiest way to help keep the vapors out of the air?

5. Why are dust masks ineffective against vapors?

6. Name five symptoms of chemical overexposure.

7. To work safely with chemicals you must lower your _____ to _____ levels.

8. What percentage of salon chemicals can never be toxic under any circumstances?

9. Are natural substances safer? Explain.

10. What should you always do before mixing, pouring, or using a liquid substance?

N I N E

Keeping Healthy Skin

Walk through any salon and look at everyone's hands. Quickly, you will discover that skin disease is a common problem. Skin disorders of the hands affects 40% of all nail technicians sometime during their careers. Skin problems are common in many occupations. In fact, skin disorders are the number one occupation-related disease in America. Many chemicals produce symptoms ranging from itchy rashes to serious burns or allergies. In this chapter you will learn how to avoid these problems and keep your skin healthy.

Skin Disease

In the salon, skin problems are usually seen on the fingers, nail beds, hands, wrists, and face. Skin disease and allergies force many good nail technicians to give up successful careers. This is especially sad, because it is completely avoidable. No one should suffer from any work-related skin disorder.

Remember the "Overexposure Principle"? It says, "Every chemical substance has a safe and unsafe level of exposure. Simply touching, inhaling, or smelling a potentially hazardous substance can't harm you. Exceeding the safe level of exposure is the danger you must learn to avoid." This important rule applies for skin disease, as well. Since so many nail technicians develop skin disease, it is tempting to blame the products. However, manufacturing workers who make and package these products rarely develop the problems seen on nail technicians! Manufacturing workers are exposed to both the concentrated raw ingredients and finished products, but manage to avoid skin problems. This is positive proof that the Overexposure

Principle is at work. Repeated overexposure and abuse are clearly the reasons nail technicians have problems.

Dermatitis

Dermatitis means skin inflammation. There are many kinds of dermatitis, but only one is important in the salon. Contact dermatitis is the most common skin disease for nail technicians. **Contact dermatitis** is caused by touching certain substances to the skin. This type of dermatitis can be acute (short term) or chronic (long term). Contact dermatitis can have several causes. The skin may be irritated by a substance. This is called irritant contact dermatitis. It is also possible to become allergic to an ingredient in a product. This is called allergic contact dermatitis.

Irritant Contact Dermatitis

Irritating substances create this skin condition. Certain chemicals will damage the dermis and epidermis. When damage occurs, the immune system springs into action. It floods the tissue with water, trying to dilute the irritating substance before it can cause more problems. This is why swelling occurs. The body is trying to stop things from getting any worse. The immune system also releases **histamines** which enlarge the blood vessels around the injury. Blood can then rush to the scene more quickly. Blood carries many things which will destroy or remove the irritating material. You can see and feel all the extra blood under the skin. The entire area becomes red, warm, and may throb. The histamines cause the itchy feeling that often accompanies contact dermatitis. After everything calms down, the swelling will go away. The surrounding skin is often left damaged and becomes scaly, cracked, and dry.

Corrosives are substances which cause rapid and sometimes irreversible skin damage. They damage the skin with painful burns which slowly heal. An example of a corrosive substance is methacrylic acid nail primers. Serious corrosive injuries must be treated immediately by a physician.

Corrosives create immediate damage, but most salon irritants require prolonged or repeated contact. Irritants usually take 24 hours or less to damage the skin. Generally, the damage is restricted to the contact area. Eliminating the irritating substance will make the symptoms disappear. If proper medical attention is received, the healing process will be accelerated and there is less chance of permanent damage or scarring.

Surprisingly, tap water is a very common salon irritant. Hands that remain damp for long periods often become sore, cracked, and chapped. Avoiding the problem is simple. Always completely dry the hands. Use moisturizing hand creams often to compensate for loss of skin oils. Frequent hand washing, especially in hard water, can further damage the skin. Cleansers and detergents worsen the problem. They increase damage by stripping away sebum and other natural skin chemicals. Prolonged or repeated contact with many solvents will strip away skin oils, leaving it dry or damaged. Sometimes it is difficult to determine the cause of the irritation. One way to identify the irritant is by observing the location of the reaction. Symptoms are always isolated to the contact area. The cause will be something that you are doing to this part of the skin.

Strong acid or alkaline solutions affect the skin's pH. Normal skin has a tremendous ability to "neutralize" solutions of different pH. Harsh alkaline and acid products overcome the skin's defenses and cause tissue damage. Phenolic disinfectants, for example, have very high pH values. These usually are in excess of pH 11. Prolonged or repeated contact with these disinfectants can overwhelm the skin's defenses and corrode the tissue. Remember, failing to follow manufacturer's warnings and instructions can mean trouble. Most (responsible) disinfectant manufacturers warn against skin contact.

Methacrylic acid primers are especially corrosive to tissue. These primers can cause serious burns if not treated with caution. Skin contact should always be avoided. Should accidental contact occur, immediately wash the area with plenty of cold water and soap. Soap is alkaline and will help neutralize the acid. Cold water will cool the area. If skin redness persists or there is an obvious burn, see a doctor. The damage may worsen if not properly treated. If primer is spilled on the clothing, remove the clothing immediately. Don't put it back on until it has been thoroughly washed. If splashed in the eyes, quick action is required. Flood the eyes with cold water while holding the eyelids open. If your salon has a wash basin with a flexible hose, use it! Continue to flood them for at least 15 minutes. Don't wait. Call a doctor immediately.

Allergic Contact Dermatitis

Nail technicians are often surprised when they or their clients become allergic to nail enhancement or other cosmetic products. Actually, this is far more common than generally believed. Studies show that allergic contact dermatitis accounts for approximately 80% of all cosmetic related skin problems. Allergic reactions occur when a person becomes sensitized to a product ingredient. **Sensitization** is an exaggerated reaction to a particular chemical. It is also called hypersensitivity.

Everyone is familiar with poison ivy allergy. About 75% of the population is allergic to this plant. Allergic reactions caused by salon products are very similar.

Allergies do not suddenly develop. It may take months or even years to become allergic to a product. The usual cause is prolonged or repeated contact. This process is called **sensitization.** The substance which causes the allergy is called a **sensitizer** or **allergen.**

Allergic contact dermatitis is much like irritant dermatitis. Many of the same things occur, (*i.e.,* redness, swelling, itching, etc.). However, it is very different in one important way. Irritations and their symptoms go away once overexposure stops. Not so with allergic reactions. Once you are sensitized, it is for life! The reason for this difference is in what your body "thinks" is happening. Some chemicals fool the immune system into thinking they are invaders, such as viruses or bacteria.

The immune system is like a great army. This massive fighting force is able to wage a full-scale war against any foreign aggressor. This army has privates and generals, spies and assassins, sentries and scouts. When it detects invaders, the immune system springs into action. Certain parts of the immune system act as spies. They rush to the area where the unknown substance is reported. The immune spies memorize the molecule and describe it in messages they send back to the generals. The generals send messengers to alert the immune system army of a possible invasion. They also describe the molecule so the army knows what to watch for. The rest of the immune system builds up its defenses and patiently waits for the attack. The immune system is ready now and stays on the lookout. If skin contact is made again, the immune system is ready and waiting. When the body reacts this way it is called an immune response.

Potent sensitizers, like poison ivy, trigger immune responses after just one exposure. Fortunately, salon product manufacturers are very careful to avoid using potent sensitizers. Most monomers and oligomers used in nail enhancement products are weak sensitizers. It is impossible to become allergic to a product after only one exposure. Rarely will it occur after several exposures. Sensitization to nail enhancement products typically takes *four to six months of repeated contact.* However, some people go years before becoming allergic. Once allergic, any contact will cause symptoms within 48 hours. These symptoms will worsen with each continued exposure.

Causes of Allergic Reactions

Determining the cause of the allergic reaction can be tricky. Unlike irritant contact dermatitis, the symptoms are not restricted to the contact area. Sometimes, swelling and other signs may occur far from the point of contact, (*i.e.*, face, armpits, and glands in the throat or groin). Also, the first signs of an allergic reaction occurs after many months of overexposure. Nail technicians are fooled into believing it was something recent which caused the reaction.

The source of an allergic reactions is easier to track down, if you know what to look for. In the early stages, tiny water blisters are often seen around the cuticle or fingertip. This is almost always caused by repeated soft tissue contact. Eventually, the symptoms worsen. They may develop into open sores. The fingertips might become numb or feel itchy under the nail plate. Continued use sometimes results in permanent loss of the nail plate.

Gels and wraps as well as monomer-polymer nail enhancements, can all cause allergic reactions. Monomers and oligomers must NEVER contact any skin, including your own. Not even once! NEVER! Unfortunately, it is easier to slop on product than it is to leave an 1/8-inch margin between product and the cuticle. Nail technicians get into the habit of touching the skin. It doesn't seem to have any immediate effect. They don't realize that they are slowly sensitizing their clientele.

Overmanicuring the cuticle can make clients more susceptible as well. Previously irritated, broken, or damaged skin increases the chance of developing an allergy. The skin is a barrier. If that barrier is broken, the risks for allergic reactions increase. It is your professional duty to avoid skin contact at all costs! This cannot be overemphasized. Nail enhancement products and chemistry cannot advance until nail technicians accept this responsibility. Many high-tech ingredients cannot be used in products because nail technicians, in general, are far too careless with their chemical tools.

The second-biggest reason for allergic reactions is using too wet a consistency. Monomer and polymer products must be used with a medium-wet consistency. Wetter ratios may help smooth the surface, but the product is difficult to control and can run into the cuticles. The initiator in the polymer powder is balanced. There is just enough initiator to react all of the monomer. Going too wet throws off this balance. A large percentage of monomer becomes trapped in the nail enhancement. This monomer eventually works its way down to the nail bed and causes an allergic reaction. It may be quicker and easier to go wetter, but in the long run both you and your client will pay the price. Extra-large or oversize brushes make overly wet beads. The belly of these large brushes can carry enough liquid for *four* normal-size beads. Brushes that are too large don't save time—they cause allergic reactions. Refer to Chapter 6 for more information on controlling consistency.

Another common reason for sensitivity to monomer-polymer systems is mixing product lines. Monomer liquids are designed to efficiently react with a specific polymer powder. Upset this delicate balance and you are asking for trouble. It may leave a high percentage of unreacted monomer trapped inside the enhancement. The excess monomer makes the enhancement look clearer and more flexible, but don't be fooled. This trap catches many nail technicians. Eventually, the excess monomer soaks through the nail plate and into the nail bed where it may sit for weeks. This "prolonged exposure" is one of the leading causes of itchy nail beds and other adverse skin reactions.

Why Risk it?

Developing a nail enhancement product takes years of experience and testing. Making new, previously unknown discoveries requires a high-tech laboratory and sophisticated chemical instruments. It is highly unlikely that anyone will "accidentally" stumble across a better mixture. It just doesn't happen that way. If you mix product lines, you may find something that looks whiter or pinker or clearer or seems more flexible. So what? Without extensive testing you can't know if there are long-term, negative side effects. If problems develop what do you do? Where can you go for help?

Imagine for a moment that you are being sued by a client who lost all of her natural nails and says it is your fault. If you are a good nail technician and follow instructions, a responsible manufacturer and any expert would testify on your behalf. You followed the instructions, so you could not be at fault. Now imagine the same situation, but the technician mixes two different polymer powders and two different monomers to create her own "secret" blend. She didn't follow instructions. No, she had her own "special" technique. What will the manufacturers and experts say about that? What *can* they say? She is probably negligent and liable for her actions. Can she justify her actions in a court of law?

Creating a new blend may seem fun and exciting (most nail technicians have a little bit of a chemist inside them), but seriously, why bother? If you don't like the product the way it is, change to another and another, until you find one that meets your expectations. Don't jeopardize yourself or your client. Follow instructions and *never* mix products or make your own blends.

Once a client becomes allergic, things will only get worse if you continue using the same products and techniques. It is best to discontinue use and figure out what you are doing wrong before more clients are affected. Somewhere, behind EVERY allergic reaction to nail products, is a careless nail technician. Don't let that nail technician be you! If your client becomes allergic to the product, you probably have

---

- NEVER go back and smooth the surface with more monomer.

- NEVER use monomer to "clean" around the edges, under the nail, or sidewalls.

- NEVER touch any monomer or oligomer to the skin (including gels and wraps).

- NEVER apply product to a client experiencing a skin reaction.

- NEVER touch the hairs of the brush with your fingers.

- NEVER mix your own product blends.

- ALWAYS follow instructions.

---

yourself to blame. Medications, illness, and other allergies don't make clients sensitive to nail products. These are just excuses. Only prolonged and repeated contact causes these allergies. Many times, clients with skin reaction or nail infection will insist that you continue to apply product. If you do so, it is at *your* own risk. You are legally responsible for your client's safety. Even if they sign a waiver or release form, you can be sued for negligence. It is your duty to refuse and discontinue use. Refer the client to a physician or dermatologist for advice. Don't try to "fix" the problem yourself. Only a qualified medical doctor is allowed to treat or cure diseased or infected skin or fingernails.

Protect Yourself

Take extreme care to keep brush handles, containers, and tabletops clean and free from product residue. Repeatedly handling these items will cause overexposure if they are not kept clean. A common area for allergies and irritation is between the thumb and forefinger. Stroking the brush hairs or cleaning the brushes with bare fingers is repeated contact. Enhancement products are not designed for skin contact! If you avoid contact, neither you or your client will ever develop an allergic reaction.

Also, avoid touching your face. Dusts and product residues can cause blemishes and skin inflammation. The cheeks are especially prone to allergy.

Another source of overexposure is table towels. Technicians often wipe brushes on a table towel, which stays on the table. Resting the arm or hand on the contaminated towel will increase the risk of sensitization. Dusts on the tabletop can do the same. Never allow your arm to rest in filings. Using too wet a consistency will make dusts which are rich in monomer residues. This can lead to sensitization, especially if the dusts are from UV gel enhancements. Many UV and visible-light gels leave a tacky, gooey film on the surface. You learned in Chapter 6 that this film is rich in unreacted oligomer. Repeated skin contact with this gooey layer can cause sensitization.

Many serious problems can be related to the above. Don't fall into these traps. Some of these bad habits are ghosts from the early years of the nail industry when there was no proper education. Don't be a victim of past mistakes and myths. Sensitization poses a special threat to nail technicians. Allergic reactions have forced an untold number of nail technicians to leave the profession.

Gloves

Keeping your skin clean will prevent irritations, allergies, and related diseases. Wearing gloves is an excellent way to lower skin exposure. There are many bad excuses for not wearing gloves, but no good reasons. "They're too uncomfortable" or "it's inconvenient" are the common excuses. Sure, wearing gloves may seem uncomfortable and inconvenient. But even your shoes would be uncomfortable if you weren't used to wearing them all the time. Once you get in the habit of wearing gloves, you won't want to work without them. Painful rashes, blisters, open sores, and cracked, dry skin are even more uncomfortable. The health risks can be inconvenient, too, especially if you develop extreme sensitivities to salon chemicals and must leave the profession. Wearing gloves is far less "inconvenient" than finding a new line of work! Once you get in the habit of wearing gloves, you'll feel uncomfortable without them. There are no good reasons for not working safely, only silly and dangerous excuses.

Today, hundreds of different types of gloves are available in dozens of materials. There are gloves that reach the shoulders, individual finger gloves, and everything in-between. You can choose powdered or powder-free, cotton-lined or unlined, straight or naturally curved fingers, ultra-sheer to heavy duty. Some gloves even have a rough texture for improved grip and handling. Above is a short list of gloves that are useful in the salon environment.

Material Type	Benefits
	Disposable Gloves
Vinyl	Inexpensive, exceptional sensitivity, and chemical resistance.
Natural Latex	Inexpensive, improved strength, good sensitivity, and chemical resistance.
Polyethylene	Lowest cost, but lower sensitivity, strength, and chemical resistance.
Polyurethane	Excellent chemical resistance and strength; tough, sheer, and high sensitivity.
	Reusable Gloves
Nitrile	Exceptional chemical resistance and strength; lower sensitivity (both disposable and reusable are available).
PVA	Exceptional chemical resistance and strength; lower sensitivity, lighter than most.
Neoprene	Good chemical resistance and strength; improved sensitivity, and flexible.

Disposable gloves should be thrown away after each use. The reusable gloves should be disposed of on the first day of each month, so you don't use them for too long. Eventually, chemicals will soak through to the inside and contaminate the skin. Try different types of gloves. That is a good way to determine which is right for you.

Allergic to Gloves?

It seems strange that a person could be allergic to wearing gloves, but it happens. This most often occurs with powdered gloves. Cornstarch is used as the powder. Powdered gloves are easier to put on or remove and they keep hands dry. A small percentage of wearers are sensitive to cornstarch. They must wear powder-free gloves. Others are sensitive to latex. It is believed that the stabilizers in latex gloves cause problems for some individuals. If you experience problems wearing any glove, consult the manufacturer or distributor. They can suggest alternative materials that will not cause problems. Whatever gloves you choose, be sure to wear them!

Nail Infections

Prevention is the only way technicians can "treat" nail infections. Nail technicians are not qualified to diagnose or treat ANY nail infection. If you attempt to treat an infected nail you are taking a major risk. Not only can you lose your license, you may be sued. Only medical doctors are licensed to treat nail infections. Recently, the FDA released a directive which forbids the sale of any product claiming to cure or prevent nail fungal infections. A team of medical experts determined that no over-the-counter medication or product can completely cure nail infections. Any apparent cure is temporary at best. In fact, it is illegal for manufacturers to make claims that imply their product may cure any fungal infection.

Unfortunately, there is no easy solution to nail infections. Doctors know almost nothing about the professional nail industry. When they see a nail infection under a nail enhancement they often react out of ignorance. They usually tell the client to take off the enhancements. They don't know what else to do. It is up to you to prevent this. Contact a local dermatologist and explain that you are a responsible and safety-conscious professional. Offer to send him or her clients that have problems. Before you do, however, make sure the dermatologist is responsible, as well. Find out what he or she knows about the nail industry and offer any information that is lacking. If you work with your local dermatologist, everyone will benefit. The doctor will learn about your profession, your clients will get proper treatment, and you will be protected from legal action.

■ FAST TRACK

- Skin disorders of the hands affect 40% of all nail technicians during their careers.

- Skin disorders are the number one occupation-related disease in America.

- Manufacturing workers who make these products rarely develop skin problems.

- Repeated overexposure and abuse is clearly the cause of salon-related skin disease.

- *Dermatitis* means skin inflammation.

- Contact dermatitis is the most common skin disease for nail technicians.

- When skin is irritated by a substance it is called irritant contact dermatitis.

- Allergic reactions are called allergic contact dermatitis.

- Irritants usually take 24 hours or less to damage the skin.

- Tap water is a very common salon irritant.

- Frequent hand washing (especially in hard water) can damage the skin.

- Strongly acid or alkaline solutions affect the skin's pH.

- Methacrylic acid primers are highly corrosive to tissue.

- Allergic contact dermatitis accounts for approximately 80% of all cosmetic-related skin problems.

- Allergic reactions occur when a person becomes sensitized to a product ingredient.

- Sensitization or hypersensitivity is an exaggerated reaction to a chemical.

- A substance which causes allergy is called a sensitizer or allergen.

- Once you are sensitized to an ingredient, it is for life!

- Most monomers and oligomers used in nail enhancement products are weak sensitizers.

- It is impossible to become allergic to a product after only one exposure.

- Sensitization to nail enhancement products takes four to six months of repeated contact.

- Monomers and oligomers must NEVER contact any skin, including your own.

- Previously irritated, broken, or damaged skin increases the chance of allergy.

- The number two reason for allergic reactions is using too wet a consistency.

- Monomer-and-polymer products must be at a medium-wet consistency.

- Using extra large or oversize brushes cause overly wet beads.

- The belly of large brushes can carry enough liquid for *four* normal-size beads.

- NEVER go back and smooth the surface with more monomer.

- NEVER use monomer to "clean" around the edges, under the nail, or sidewalls.

- NEVER touch any monomer or oligomer to the skin (including gels and wraps).

- NEVER apply product to a client experiencing a skin reaction.

- NEVER touch the hairs of the brush with your fingers.

- NEVER mix your own product blends.

- ALWAYS follow instructions.

- Keep brush handles, containers, and tabletops clean and free of product residue.

- Dusts and product residues can cause facial blemishes and skin inflammation.

- Resting the arm or hand on a contaminated towel increases the risk of sensitization.

- Never allow your arm to rest in dusts or filings.

- Wearing gloves is an excellent way to lower skin exposure.

- Disposable gloves should be thrown away after each use.

- Reusable gloves should be disposed of once a month.

- A small percentage of wearers are sensitive to cornstarch found inside disposable gloves.

- Stabilizers in latex gloves cause sensitivities in some individuals.

- Whatever gloves you choose, be sure to wear them!

Questions

Chapter 9

1. What is the most common occupational disease in America?

2. Which is more dangerous to the skin: irritants or corrosives? Why?

3. What is the difference between an irritant and a sensitizer?

4. Name two common salon irritants.

5. Define sensitization.

6. Name five types of glove materials.

7. Most monomers and oligomers used in nail enhancement products are _____ sensitizers.

8. The substance which causes the allergy is called a _____ or _____.

9. What is the best way to avoid allergic reactions and irritations?

T E N

Improving Your Air Quality

"Use Adequate Ventilation!" We see this familiar warning almost everywhere. What is "adequate ventilation" anyway? How do I know if my salon has proper ventilation? What are the consequences of ignoring these warnings? In this chapter you will learn what proper ventilation is and isn't. You will also see that proper ventilation offers great advantages and benefits.

Odors

Why use ventilation? People generally believe ventilation is used to reduce odors. Many believe that odors are dangerous and must be eliminated. As you learned in the last chapter, this is a common misconception in the nail industry. This foolish myth implies that odor determines the safety of a chemical. Many wrongly think that products with sweet, pleasant aromas must contain good, wholesome ingredients. Who would think they needed ventilation if the room smelled nice? It is our animal nature to be attracted to nice smells and to be suspicious of strange or funny odors. We assume that chemicals which smell bad must be dangerous. Nothing could be further from the truth! Odor is caused by vapors stimulating the nerves in our nose. It has nothing to do with chemical safety. Does your kidney or liver care what the products smell like? Of course not! Odors *are* useful. Odors help determine if the salon environment is safe.

How's the Air?

First we must decide if our salon environment needs improvement. The following checklist will help rate the quality of your breathing air.

- Do strong product odors linger for more than ten minutes?

- Can strong odors be detected far away from the source, (*i.e.,* the other side of the salon)?

- Do you still smell product odors when you open the shop in the morning?

- Do the walls ever "sweat" with moisture or the windows become foggy?

- Do clients complain of offensive odors?

- Do you ever have to open the window or door because the odors become too strong?

- Do any employees *frequently* complain of one or more of the following symptoms: headaches, nausea, sore throats, coughs, blurry vision, watery eyes, insomnia, irritability, drowsiness, dizziness, runny or bloody noses, sneezing, tingling toes or fingers, chest aches or pains, shortness of breath and/or loss of coordination or appetite?

- Do you find that strong odors don't bother you anymore or that you just don't smell them?

- Do you get funny tastes in your mouth or does food lack flavor?

The last two bulleted points may seem unrelated, but these are two important warning signs of improper ventilation. Some nail technicians consider themselves lucky because they don't even notice product odors. They are suffering from **olfactory fatigue**. In other words, the olfactory gland (your nose) has gotten tired of the overwhelming smell. It just quits smelling it! Unfortunately, this can result in permanent damage and may drastically reduce your ability to smell. Once this happens, you will also lose the ability to properly taste food. Imagine for the rest of your life, chocolate cake tasting bland!

If you answered yes to even *one* of the questions above then your ventilation could stand improvement. This checklist shows how odors can help determine air quality. Odors are tools, not the enemy. Well then, why use ventilation? In Chapter 8 you learned that there are three types of air contaminants:

- Vapors

- Mists

- Dusts

Each of these may increase the risks of overexposure if they are not controlled. Vapors come from the evaporation of liquids. Mists are fine droplets of liquid created by aerosol and pump sprayers. Dust particles ranging from the very large (pinhead-size) to invisible, microscopic particles. Luckily, these air contaminants are easily controlled. It is possible to "breathe easy" in the salon and protect your health – if you know how.

Breathing Zones

Every one is concerned about the environment. Protecting the quality of our air is vital. Still, there is one place on Earth that is more important to you than any other. That place is called your **breathing zone.** Your breathing zone is an invisible sphere about twice the size of a basketball. It sits directly in front of your mouth. You can't see it, but it is always there. When you turn your head or leave the room, your breathing zone moves with you. Every single breath you take in your life comes from your breathing zone. Fewer things have a greater impact on your health than what occurs in this small area. There can be no better reason to protect this precious space. This is the true purpose of ventilation.

Proper ventilation protects your breathing zone.

Excessive inhalation of vapors is a problem for nail technicians. These vapors come from the evaporation of liquids. It is a common myth that certain liquids do not evaporate. This is false! All liquid nail products evaporate and contribute to the total vapors in the air. Odorless monomers and gel oligomers are good examples. Some believe that the lower odor of these products means they no longer need to worry about proper ventilation. Just because you can't smell anything doesn't mean your air is clean. All vapors, with or without odors, must be controlled if you are to protect your salon environment. The same is true for pleasant fragrances. Spraying perfumes or using aromatherapy or scented nail products can be dangerous. These are only cover-ups. Covering odors is not the answer. This can actually increase your chance of vapor overexposure. This is akin to closing your eyes when you cross the street. Just because you don't see the cars doesn't mean they aren't there.

What can you do to lower your exposure to vapors? Luckily, some of the most effective ways to eliminate vapors are the easiest and least expensive.

1. Keep all products tightly sealed when not in use.

Any liquid product will create vapors. It may be more convenient to leave the cap off, but it will certainly increase your risks. Leaving containers open can ruin your product's effectiveness. This unsafe practice also drastically increases the danger of accidental spills.

2. Use a covered dappen dish.

Monomer liquids must be easily accessible. It isn't practical to keep monomer in a sealed container while using the product. However, you can keep the monomer in a dappen dish with lid. Many dishes have covers with holes in the center. Use a marble to cover the hole in your dappen dish cover. *Never* use a dappen dish without a lid.

3. Avoid pressurized spray containers.

Pressurized spray cans create much finer mists which are difficult to control. Avoid pressurized cans. If you can use a pump sprayer, you will eliminate a potential source of overexposure.

4. Empty your waste container often.

Waste containers are one of the best sources of vapors. If you wipe up a spill and then throw it into the trash, those vapors will soon be in your breathing zone. Metal waste containers with pop-up lids are great for controlling vapors. Remember to empty your trash several times each day and before you leave at night. Good housekeeping is an important safety tool.

5. Don't wipe dirty brushes on your table towel.

Most nail enhancement monomers are very volatile. They will quickly evaporate. Wiping your brush on a towel is the same as putting that chemical into the air. Use a disposable wipe and throw it away. Remember, avoid skin contact with anything you use to wipe your brush.

These five simple steps can dramatically improve the quality of your salon air, but you must do more. Your salon still must be properly ventilated.

What to Avoid!

There is so much incorrect information about ventilation that nail technicians frequently do the wrong things. Let's explore the facts of ventilation. Then, making the proper choice will be easy.

FACT: Proper salon ventilation doesn't circulate air.

Open doors, windows, air conditioners, and fans are not ventilation–they are *circulation*. These methods circulate the vapors around the room so everyone can breathe them equally! High-quality ventilation systems do not just spread vapors around the room.

FACT: Ventilation systems do not "purify the air".

It is possible to purify the air. Devices in the space shuttle purify the air for the astronauts. However, you can bet that NASA didn't pay $800 for the system! It is IMPOSSIBLE to purify the air in a salon. Installing such a device in the salon would cost a tremendous amount of money. Luckily, it isn't necessary to purify the air. Remember the "Overexposure Principle"? You need only to lower your exposure to a safe level. Never buy a device which claims to purify the air. You will be disappointed.

FACT: Don't ventilate odors

Many devices sold to nail technicians and salon owners claim that they eliminate odors. As you have learned, eliminating odors doesn't mean the air is clean. Remember, vapors are what needs to be removed and controlled. Do this properly and there will be no odor problem. As you will see below, many devices cleverly conceal odors without removing any vapors.

Ventilated Nail Table

These tables rely on a tray filled with activated charcoal to remove the vapor. Although the theory is good, in practice they have very little effectiveness. Activated charcoal is like a chemical sponge which absorbs vapors from the air. But like a sponge, they soon become saturated and ineffective. These filters are usually lightweight and loosely filled with absorbing charcoal. You can see through many of them. Besides, monomer vapors are not easily absorbed by activated charcoal. To remain useful, these expensive filter trays must be replaced at least once a week.

Twice weekly is better! Never reuse a filter, either. Shaking out the collected nail dust does not shake out the absorbed chemicals. Once they have been used, throw them away. Does this mean you should throw out your ventilated table, too? Of course not, but don't rely solely on these tables to protect your salon environment.

Ozone Generators

Ozone generators are sold as devices which remove odors. Some manufacturers try to fool nail technicians. They claim that ozone will change salon vapors to harmless carbon dioxide, air, and water. The advertisements boast that ozone changes dangerous chemicals to a harmless state. It would be wonderful if this were really true! Factories would simply mount ozone generators on their smoke stacks and our nation's air pollution problem would disappear. Of course, this is as silly as it sounds. Ozone can do this only under special laboratory conditions not found in the the real world. In the salon, ozone does change vapors. Ozone converts the vapors into different substances, usually with a lower or different odor. However, there are just as many vapors as before; only now you don't know they are there. Also, the new vapor may be even more harmful to breathe. No one really knows! Ozone is also a major component in smog. High concentrations of ozone can be hazardous to your health and may cause eye, throat, and lung irritation. These devices are not useful in the salon environment.

HEPA Filters

HEPA filters are High Efficiency Particle Filters. They are extremely good at capturing dusts, but they have no effect on vapors. Vapor molecules are hundreds of times smaller than dust particles. They whiz right through a HEPA filter. Devices that filter dust from the air have absolutely no effect on vapors. Some HEPA filters are used in combination with high quality, activated charcoal filters. Densely packed charcoal filters can absorb vapors for up to four months. However, even these devices are not useful in the salon.

Ventilation MUST protect your breathing zone. The best HEPA filter can't protect your breathing zone as efficiently as a simple dust mask! Why? HEPA filters sit on a table in the corner of a room. Even if placed by your station, they can't outperform a ten-cent dust mask. When you file, the highest concentration of dust in the room is between your mouth and the client's hand. HEPA filters can help remove dusts from the room, but dust masks filter your breathing air! In the long run, masks are the best way to reduce exposure to dust. HEPA filters are useful in the salon, but they don't eliminate the need for dust masks. Use both for optimum protect from dust inhalation.

Ionizers

Ionizers are devices which create ions. These ions put a static-like charge on dust particles. Once charged, dust particles clump together into microscopic clusters. The large clusters then fall from the air. Ionizers can also make the air appear to smell "fresh," like after a rainstorm. This is because nature often produces ions after it rains. But, knocking a dust particle from the air doesn't remove it from the salon. Also, ionizers provide no breathing zone protection and they have NO effect on vapors.

Absorber Units

Absorbers are units which are usually placed on the nail table. They contain substances that are supposed to attract vapors or odors and absorb them. These units are extremely ineffective in salons. Despite the claims, they can only absorb a tiny percentage of the vapors in the salon air. They work best in small, enclosed areas with musty, damp smells. They can also remove cigarette odors. They may work well for the home, but these units can't possibly keep up with all the vapors generated in the salon. Only a tiny fraction of the vapors in the salon find there way into the unit to be absorbed. It would take dozens of these units to have even a moderate effect on the salon air and they would have to be changed weekly. In short, they are not suited for the salon environment. As with many other devices, they are sold as odor removers. Remember, devices which only *remove* odors don't make the salon air any safer.

Ventilated tables, ionizers, absorbers, and ozone generators are not practical for the salon. HEPA filters are designed to work on the entire salon environment, not your breathing zone. Well then, what's a safety-conscious nail technician to do about ventilation? What is the best way to get rid of vapors?

Local Exhaust

The only complete answer to salon vapor control is **local exhaust.** These devices are based on a simple concept. They capture the vapors at the source and expel them from your breathing zone. Local exhaust uses an exhaust vent, hose, or tube to capture vapors, dusts, and mists. A movable exhaust tube can be placed where needed, (*i.e.,* over your open containers or beside the hand while you file). Specially designed blowers pull contaminants from the breathing zone, down the exhaust tube, and expel them from the building.

Although venting to the outside is preferred, it is not always possible. If your salon has no outside access, the vapors and dusts can be filtered through a HEPA filter and a five-gallon canister packed with activated charcoal. If you can vent to the roof, make sure your exhaust pipe is at least 15 feet from any intake vents, especially your neighbors'. The higher it is above the roof, the better. This will prevent odors from being drawn into nearby homes or businesses.

Local exhaust is by far the easiest and in the long run, least expensive solution. Presently, only one company supplies a ready-made system which is useful in salons. Lab Safety Supply sells a local exhaust system that is fairly easy to install and highly effective in the salon environment. It is also very attractive, with a high-tech look that will appeal to clients. The two devices they sell are called the Fume Extractor and Fume Vac. Either system is ideal for salons. You can reach Lab Safety Supply at 1-800-356-2501. Ask for a free copy of their latest general catalog. It contains many useful items ranging from dust and mist masks to gloves and safety glasses. They also have a technical help line that can answer many of your safety-related questions.

Another alternative is to have a local ventilation expert custom design a system. Custom systems can be built fairly inexpensively. Have them design a system similar to the Lab Safety's Fume Vac. An expert capable of building such a system is as close as your phone book. Look under Heating or Air Conditioning for a specialist that understands proper ventilation. You'll be surprised at how affordable a well-designed local ventilation system can be.

Properly designed systems capture vapors, mists, and dusts at the source and remove them before they can enter your breathing zone or salon environment. You will be amazed the first time you see a large dust particle fall from your file, make a U-turn in the air, and disappear into the exhaust vent! It is best to use a movable tube to capture the contaminants. Air flow should not pull vapors past your face but, instead, away from you. Also, the system should be capable of capturing between 50-100 feet per minute (fpm) of air. A well-designed system is extremely efficient and can actually save money on your heating and air conditioning bill.

Of course, no system is completely foolproof. There is no magic cure-all. You must still do everything you can to protect your salon environment from vapors and other chemical contamination. As you learned in other chapters, there is no substitute for a well-fitting, disposable dust mask. You must follow all the other recommended procedures to minimize vapors in the salon. Overexposure can occur in many ways. Working safely means always being on the lookout for ways to reduce exposure.

Your clients will love to see you taking safety precautions. It will give them more confidence in your knowledge and ability. Remember to teach them about the Overexposure Principle. Reassure them that they run little risk of becoming over-exposed. They'll be relieved to see that you are safety aware.

Before You Go – A Final Reminder

Let the Overexposure Principle guide you throughout your career. It is possible to use professional nail products without fear or apprehension, but chemical safety doesn't just happen. It takes effort and attention. Always look for techniques and products which lower your exposure. This is the key to working safely. This is also the key to chemical awareness and understanding. With this knowledge you will join the ranks of the modern, "chemically aware" nail technician. Good luck, good health, and please.... be safe!

FAST TRACK

- Nail technicians who can't smell strong odors are suffering from olfactory fatigue.
- Olfactory fatigue may permanently affect the sense of smell and taste.
- The three types of air contaminants are vapors, mists, and dusts.
- The most important place on Earth should be your breathing zone.
- Your breathing zone is an invisible sphere about twice the size of a basketball.
- Proper ventilation protects your breathing zone.
- Vapors come from the evaporation of liquids.
- All vapors, with or without odors, must be controlled.
- Perfumes, aromatherapy, or scented nail products can increase exposure to vapors.
- Keep all products tightly sealed when not in use.
- Use a covered dappen dish.
- Keep the monomer in a dappen dish with a lid.
- Avoid pressurized spray containers.
- Empty your waste container often.

- Don't wipe dirty brushes on your table towel.

- Avoid skin contact with anything you use to wipe your brush.

- Proper salon ventilation doesn't circulate air.

- Ventilation systems do not "purify the air."

- Don't ventilate odors.

- Don't rely on these ventilated nail tables to protect your salon environment.

- Ozone CANNOT neutralize or remove salon vapors.

- High concentrations of ozone can be hazardous to your health.

- HEPA filters are High Efficiency Particle Filters.

- HEPA filters have no effect on vapors.

- Ventilation MUST protect your breathing zone.

- Ionizers provide no breathing zone protection and have NO effect on vapors.

- The only complete answer to salon vapor control is local exhaust.

- If you vent to the roof, make sure your exhaust pipe is at least 15 feet from any intake vent.

- Your ventilation system should be capable of capturing between 50-100 feet per minute (fpm) of air.

- Please.... be safe!

Questions

Chapter 10

1. _____ is when your nose can no longer smell a strong odor.

2. Your _____ is an invisible sphere about twice the size of a basketball.

3. Never use a _____ without a lid.

4. What is the most important job of a good ventilation system?

5. What are the risks of using ozone generators?

6. Why are HEPA filters unable to capture vapors?

7. What is local exhaust?

8. A good local exhaust system must capture between ___–___ fpm of air.

9. If you vent to the salon's roof, the exhaust pipe should be at least _____ from any intake vent.

10. _____ is like a chemical sponge.

Appendix

Glossary

NOTE: This glossary defines the technical words used in this book which appear in **boldface.** Many of these words have multiple meanings. The definitions given are those related to the subjects discussed in this book. For other definitions, consult a dictionary, encyclopedia, or other reference material. Call your local library for assistance.

Acrylates – Family of monomers used in light-curing gel products.

Acute hepatitis – Liver inflammation lasting for several weeks or months.

Acute – Short-term.

Adhesion – A force of nature that makes two surfaces stick together when the molecules on one surface are attracted to the molecules on another surface.

Adhesive – A chemical that causes two surfaces to stick together.

Adhesive bond – The area between two adhered surfaces.

Allergen – A substance that causes an allergy.

Amino acids – Small chemicals which the body uses to build proteins.

Antiseptic – Sanitizers which help prevent skin infections.

Arteries – Tubes that carry blood from the heart to other parts of the body.

Bacterial spores – A dormant state of some bacteria. Spores can become active, living bacteria under the correct conditions. Spores are the most rugged and resistant form of life known.

Bactericides – Substances which kill harmful bacteria.

Beading – Caused when liquids are repelled by a solid surface.

Benzoyl peroxide – Heat-sensitive initiator used in two-part, monomer-and-polymer nail enhancement systems.

Bilirubin – A pigment which is quickly broken down by normal, healthy livers.

Breathing zone – An invisible two-foot sphere extending outward from your mouth and containing all your breathing air.

Brittleness – A property of a substance that determines how likely it is to break if force is applied.

Capillaries – Small branches that carry blood to and from the nail unit or other cells.

Carpel tunnel – A small passage in a wrist bone which houses a nerve that runs from the fingers into the arm.

Carpel tunnel syndrome – See Cumulative Trauma Disorder.

Carrier – A person who shows no outward symptoms of infection, but carries a communicable virus capable of infecting others.

Cell – The smallest and simplest unit capable of being alive.

Chemical – One of the building blocks of all matter. Everything can see or touch, except light and electricity, is a chemical.

Chemical change – The process of converting a chemical into an entirely different chemical substance, ie., wood burning into ashes or polymerizing monomers into a polymer.

Chemical reaction – The process of combining two or more chemicals into a new chemical substance.

Chronic – Long-term.

Chronic hepatitis – Liver inflammation lasting longer than six months.

Cirrhosis – Permanent liver scarring.

Co- – Two or more working together.

Coatings – Products which cover the nail plate with a hard film.

Consistency – The ratio of monomer-to-polymer.

Contact Dermatitis – Skin inflammation caused by touching certain substances to the skin.

Contaminant – Substance which causes contamination.

Contamination – Foreign substances on a implement or surface.

Copolymer – A polymer made from two or more different monomers.

Corrosive – A substance which causes visible and sometimes permanent damage to human skin.

Cross-linker – A monomer capable of joining different polymer chains together.

Cross-links – Chemical bonds between two protein, acrylic, or other polyme chains.

CTD – See Cumulative Trauma Disorder

Cumulative Trauma Disorder (CTD) – A number of painful and crippling illnesses caused by repetitive motion.

Cure – See polymerization.

Curing – Popular slang for any process which causes monomers to chemically react into a polymer.

Cyanoacrylates – Family of monomers used in wraps, no-light gels and instant nail adhesives.

Cystine – An amino acid which forms the sulfur cross-links in nails and hair.

Decontamination – The eliminate of pathogens or other substances from a contaminated implement or surface.

Delamination – Peeling apart of two improperly adhered surfaces.

Dermatitis – Skin inflammation.

Dermis – Basement tissue, lower layer of skin on the nail bed, farthest from the nail plate.

Disinfectants – Substances which kill all microorganisms, except bacteria spores, on nonliving surfaces.

Disinfection – The second level of decontamination. Controls microorganisms on nonliving surfaces.

Distal – "Farthest from the attached end," opposite of proximal.

Distal nail plate – The part of the nail plate which grows beyond the fingertip. Also called the free edge.

EPA – Environmental Protection Agency.

EPA registration number – A number assigned to all disinfectants registered by this agency.

Element – The smallest part that matter can be divided into without destroying it.

Epidermis – Upper-layer skin on the nail bed, closest to the nail plate.

Eponychium – The visible skin fold which appears to stop at the base of the nail plate.

Evaporation rate – A measure of how quickly a liquid will convert into a vapor at room temperature.

Exotherm – Heat released by a chemical reaction.

Exothermic – Heat releasing.

Exothermic reaction – Chemical reactions which release heat.

FDA – Food and Drug Administration.

Flexibility – A property of a substance that determines how much it will bend if a force is applied.

Flow modifier – An ingredient which reduces brush strokes on the surface.

Formaldehyde – A suspected human cancer-causing agent and poison used for many years as a salon disinfectant.

Formalin – See Formaldehyde.

Free edge – The part of the nail plate which grows beyond the fingertip. Also called the distal nail plate.

Free radicals – Very excited molecules which cause many kinds of chemical reactions.

Fumes – Tiny, solid particles suspended in smoke.

Fungicides – Substances which destroy fungus.

Gelling – Slow thickening of enhancement products in the container.

Gels – Thickened liquids. Also, UV light-curing oligomers or thickened wrap monomers.

Glass beads sterilizers – Devices which are supposed to sterilize salon implements, but are actually ineffective in the salon.

Glues – Adhesives made from protein, usually animal.

Hardness – A measure of how easily a substance is scratched or dented.

Heat-curing – Using the heat of infrared energy, to polymerize nail enhancement monomers.

Heat – See Infrared light.

Hepatitis – A general term describing any infection or inflammation (swelling) of the liver.

Hepatitis A – A viral hepatitis caused by eating food or water contaminated by feces.

Hepatitis B – A serious viral hepatitis transmitted in the exact same way as HIV. Also called serum hepatitis.

Hepatitis C – A serious form of hepatitis linked to chronic liver disease and cancer.

Homo – Means "same."

Homopolymer – A polymer made from only one type of monomer.

Hospital level – A certification assigned to disinfectants by the EPA. Shows that the disinfectant was tested and proven to be effective against specific microorganisms.

Hyponychium – The most distal edge of the nail unit and of the nail bed.

Infectious hepatitis – Also called hepatitis A.

Infrared light – Invisible light energy just below the color red. Also called heat.

Inhibitors – Ingredients which prevent monomers from joining.

Initiator – A molecule that starts polymerization by transferring stored energy to a monomer. See Polymerization.

IPNs – Abbreviation for Interpenetrating Polymer Network. Polymers which weave through another cross-linked polymer with further increasing cross-linking.

Jaundice – A symptom of many diseases including hepatitis. Causes yellowing of the eyes and skin.

Keratin – The chemical substance which makes up the nail plate. A protein made from amino acids.

Lateral – "To the side."

Lateral nail fold – The skin on either side of the nail plate. An extension of the proximal nail fold.

Light-curing – Using special lamps to polymerize nail enhancement monomers.

Local exhaust – Special ventilation that captures vapors and dust at the source and removes them from the workplace or breathing zone.

Lunula – "Half-moon"; the whitish, opaque area at the base (proximal end) of the nail plate formed by immature keratin cells.

Matrix – Small area of living tissue directly below the proximal nail fold.

Matter – The substance of which all physical things are composed.

Mer – Units.

Methacrylates – A family of monomer used in several types of nail enhancement systems.

Methyl methacrylate – A monomer no longer used by responsible manufacturers because it causes intense allergic reactions.

Micro – "Very small."

Micron – A measurement for very small items. A human hair is about 100 microns wide and a 50 micron particle is half as thick as a hair.

Microorganisms – A general term for any very tiny, microscopic living creatures.

Molecule – The basic chemical building blocks of all matter.

Mono – "One."

Monomer – "One unit or molecule." A molecule which reacts to form a polymer.

Nail bed – Lies directly under the nail plate.

Nail unit – Consists of the seven major parts of the fingernail.

Natural nail – Nail plate.

Natural nail overlays – Coatings which cover only the nail plate.

Nitrocellulose – A polymer used in the production of many nail polishes and topcoats.

No-light gel – Wraps monomers that have been thickened to have a gel-like appearance.

Odorless acrylics – A term used to describe acrylic liquids which are not easily detected by the human sense of smell. Not necessarily indicative of low evaporation rate or safeness.

Olfactory fatigue – Loss of the ability to detect certain odors due to long term overexposure. In advanced cases, a permanent loss of taste often occurs.

Oligomers – A single chain that is several thousand monomers long, but not long enough to be a polymer.

Onychodermal band – The seal between the nail plate and hyponychium.

Optical brightener – An ingredient that makes colors look brighter and whites look whiter.

Organism – Any living thing.

Parts per million (PPM) – Generally, this is a measurement of the number of molecules of a vapor found in one million molecules of air, but can also be used to measure many other things.

Pathogens – Microorganisms which cause disease.

Phenolics – A category of chemicals often used in tuberculocidal disinfectants.

Physical change – The process of converting a substance from one physical form into another, *i.e.,* a liquid into a vapor or a solid.

Plasticizers – Ingredients which improve flexibility and toughness.

Poly – "Many."

Polymerization – A chemical reaction that converts monomers into polymers.

Polymerize – See polymerization.

Polymers – "Many units or molecules." Very long chains of molecules made from monomers.

Porcelain – A term incorrectly used to describe monomer-and-polymer system.

PPM – See Parts per million.

Primers (nail plate primers) – Substances that make the nail plate more compatible to certain liquids.

Protein – Chemical substances made from long chains of amino acids.

Proximal – "Nearest attached end," opposite of distal.

Proximal nail fold – The skin fold over the part of the nail plate attached to the finger.

Quaternary ammonium compounds (quats) – A category of chemicals which are safe, effective, and low-cost salon disinfection substances.

Quats – See Quaternary ammonium compounds.

Risk assessment – Estimations of the likelihood of injury or death.

Routes of entry – The three passageways by which chemicals can enter the body: skin, mouth, and lungs.

Sanitation – To significantly reduce the numbers of pathogens from a surface to levels considered safe by public health standards.

Sanitizing – See sanitation.

Saturated – Refers to cases when a solvent has reached the maximum amount of solute it is capable of dissolving.

Sculptured nail – Coating extended past the free edge of the nail plate to form a tip.

Sensitization – Greatly increased or exaggerated sensitivity to products.

Serum hepatitis – Also called hepatitis B.

Shock curing – Overly rapid curing of a polymer. Causes thousands of microscopic cracks that make surface look cloudy white, instead of clear.

Shrinkage – Caused when billions of monomers suddenly come closer together to create a polymer that occupies less space.

Silanes – Special wetting agents that are additives that allow faster penetration of fibers.

Simple polymer chains – Uncross-linked polymers.

Solehorn or **solehorn cuticle** – Epidermis attached to the underside of the nail plate.

Solute – A substance which is dissolved in a solvent.

Solvent – A substance capable of dissolving another substance.

Spores – See Bacterial spores.

Sterilization – A process that destroys all living organisms on an object or surface.

Streaking – See Beading.

Strength – The ability of a substance to withstand breakage if force is applied.

Sulfur cross-links – Cross-links made between two cystine amino acids.

Surface – The exposed portion of a solid or liquid.

Tip and overlays – Cover an artificial tip and the natural nail plate.

Titanium dioxide – A white mineral used to create white tip powders or to give a natural appearance.

Toughness – Property of a substance that combines strength and flexibility.

True cuticle – Layer of colorless skin that is constantly shed from the underside of the proximal nail fold.

Tuberculosis – A bacterial lung disease caused by *Mycobacterium Tuberculosis*.

Ultraviolet light – The invisible energy level of light above violet.

Ultraviolet (UV) sanitizers – Implement storage containers which use UV light to keep the contents sanitized.

UV absorbers – Additives which absorb damaging UV light and act like sunscreens for enhancements.

UV light – See Ultraviolet light.

Vapor – The gaseous form of a substance that is normally a liquid at room temperature.

Vaporization – The process of converting a liquid into its gaseous state.

Vaporize – See Vaporization.

Veins – Tubes which collect blood from the capillaries and return it to the heart.

Viricides – Substances which kill viruses.

Visible light cure – A type of light-curing which uses violet and blue light as energy instead of ultraviolet light or heat.

Visible spectrum – The colors of the rainbow: red, green, orange, yellow, green, blue and violet.

Volatile – Describes a substance that is easily converted from a liquid into a vapor.

Wet sanitizers – An incorrect name for solution containers designed to disinfect implements.

Wetting – Occurs when a liquid spreads evenly over a surface without beading or streaking.

Wetting agents – Special ingredients that make liquid surfaces more compatible with solid surfaces.

Answers to Chapter Questions

Chapter 1

1. Proximal means "nearest attached end," distal means "farthest attached end," and lateral means "to the side."

2. The narrowest matrix makes the narrowest nail plate. Therefore, the little finger must have the narrowest matrix.

3. matrix

4. Matrix, proximal nail fold, lateral nail fold, nail plate, nail bed, hyponychium, eponychium, true cuticle, solehorn, onychodermal band, free edge, and lunula.

5. Arteries, veins

6. Epidermis, top layer, and dermis or basement layer, bottom layer

7. The nail plate protects the nail bed. Overfiling thins the plate so that it cannot protect the delicate matrix.

8. Keratin, found in skin and hair.

9. The hyponychium forms a protective barrier that prevents bacteria, fungi, and viruses from infecting the nail bed. An infection may lead to separation of the nail plate from the nail bed.

10. The nail bed consists of two types of tissue, epidermis and dermis. The epidermis is firmly attached to the nail plate, but has ridges that allow it to freely glide over the dermis's grooves.

Chapter 2

1. The normal thumb nail will grow about $1/10$ inch per month or $1\,1/2$ inches per year.

2. One-quarter inch.

3. No cosmetic product may claim that it will change or alter any body function in any way. Cosmetic-related products are for beautifying only, not healing. No cosmetic-related product can heal, repair, grow, or make any other similar claim.

4. Cells are the smallest and simplest units capable of being alive.

5. Keratin protein chains are tied together with sulfur cross-links made from a special type of amino acid called cystine.

6. The top surface of the free edge.

7. Strength is the ability of the nail plate to withstand breakage. Hardness measures how easily the plate is scratched or dented. Flexibility determines how much the plate will bend. Brittleness shows how likely the nail is to break if force is applied. Toughness is a combination of strength and flexibility.

8. tough or have toughness

9. the many cystine sulfur cross-links, moisture

10. dry, temporary

Chapter 3

1. Everything you can see or touch, except light and electricity (energy), is a chemical.

2. Matter occupies space and is made of chemicals, energy is not made of chemicals and doesn't take up any space.

3. A molecule is a chemical in its simplest form.

4. Vapors are formed when liquids evaporate into the air, (*i.e.,* water and solvent vapors). Fumes are solid particles mixed with smoke (*i.e.,* chimney smoke and welding fumes).

5. All odors are caused by vapors in the air, not fumes!

6. a). There are a lot of the vapor's molecules in the air, (*i.e.,* very volatile).

    b). It is because the nerves in the nose are very sensitive to the vapor molecule, even in extremely low amounts.

7. A chemical change occurs when a chemical turns into something different (i.e., sugar or paper burning). Physical change only changes the outward appearance of the chemical, (i.e., freezing water or dissolving salt).

8. A catalyst is a chemical that changes the rate of a chemical reaction. They make a nail technician's work easier and faster. For example, the chemical reactions used to make artificial nail enhancements might take months to happen without a catalyst. A catalyst reduces the time to minutes.

9. A solvent is anything which dissolves another substance. The substance being dissolved is called a solute.

10. Solvents only dissolve a certain amount of solute before they become saturated. Then the solvent can no longer dissolve solute. Using a saturated solvent wastes time and needlessly exposes the client's skin to solvents.

Chapter 4

1. Adhesion is caused when the molecules on one surface are attracted to the molecules on another surface.

2. repel

3. Wetting agents

4. The adhered interface between two surfaces is called the adhesive bond.

5. When two adhered surfaces peel away from each other it is called delamination. Properly cleaning the surface and correct application techniques will help prevent delamination.

6. adhesive

7. Glues are adhesives made from protein, usually animal. Glues are low strength and don't adhere well to the nail. Glues usually dissolve easily in water.

8. Nail plate primers make the nail plate more compatible to certain liquids. Therefore, they improve adhesion.

9. Scrubbing, properly dehydrating, and avoiding skin contact will ensure good adhesion. These steps, along with proper application technique, will prevent delamination. Roughing the plate causes dangerous and excessive thinning of the natural nail. This must be avoided at all cost.

10. Drills and heavy abrasives can heat the nail bed to over 150°F, hot enough to fry an egg! They can cause overthinning of the nail plate and may promote allergic reactions and infections.

Chapter 5

1. Coatings cover the nail plate with a hard film (i.e., nail polish, topcoats, artificial enhancements and adhesives). The two types are
   a. coatings that cure or polymerize, and
   b. coatings that harden upon evaporation

2. polymerization

3. Many monomer units, or molecules, hook together to make a long polymer chain. Each individual molecule is called a monomer. *Mono* means one. *Poly* means many and mer means units. So, polymers are made from many monomers.

4. When the head of one monomer reacts with the tail of another, this long chain of monomers makes a simple polymer chain. When many simple chains are hooked together with cross-linking monomers, a net-like structure is created. These polymers are cross-linked (like rungs on a ladder or a cargo net).

5. The surface may be hard enough to file, but it will be days before the chains reach their ultimate lengths. So, the chemical reaction (polymerization) isn't finished for quite some time.

6. Light and heat. They are the only energy useful for making nail enhancements polymers.

7. Monomers don't touch each other until they polymerize. After they polymerize they embrace each other tightly. When billions of monomers suddenly come closer together the effect is very noticeable. This is what we call shrinkage.

8. When two monomers join a small amount of heat is released. This is called an exotherm or exothermic reaction. You can't feel the heat released from two monomers, but the heat released from many billions of monomers in the nail enhancement can be quite noticeable.

9. No, they form coatings strictly by evaporation.

10. ▪ Adhere several tips to wooden pusher sticks.

    ▪ Use these to make an overlay or sculptured nail enhancement as you would usually do. (NOTE: Be sure to use a clear powder. Pink powders can cover up product discoloration.) On one tip use your old product. Place the new product on a different tip.

    ▪ Place both enhancements in direct sunlight for a few days.

    ▪ Check them each day to see which yellows first. (A properly formulated product will not yellow, even after days of exposure.)

    ▪ Repeat the test if you are still unsure. Test many products until you find the one you like.

Chapter 6

1. The acrylics.

2. UV absorbers are ingredients that prevent discoloration caused by sunlight (a major cause of yellowing). It does this by absorbing damaging UV light and changing it into blue light or heat.

3. Most polymer powder particles are around 50-100 microns (one hair thickness to one-half a hair's thickness). However, they can be as large as 125 microns or as small as 10 microns ($1/10$ of a hair's thickness).

4. Excessive monomer lowers the consistency and reduces strength. This means more breakage. The highest strength is obtained when using the correct ratio of monomer to polymer.

5. Inhibitors are ingredients which prevent polymerizations. They improve shelf life and help prevent the monomer from gelling.

6. Too wet, too large or oversized, wrong

7. The bead should melt out fairly slowly over 15 seconds. Then the bead should hold its shape. The overall height of the bead should drop a little, about $1/4$ of the original height is in the right ball park.

8. Methyl methacrylate (MMA) causes intense allergic reactions and can cause serious damage to nail plates if they are jammed.

9. Warm the remover in a bottle just large enough to hold all of the solvent needed for the job. Loosen the cap to allow vapors to escape. Place the warming bottle under a stream of hot running tap water, or in a bowl filled with hot tap water. Neither the water nor the solvent should be hotter than a Jacuzzi® (110°F maximum).

10. Call the local State Board immediately!

Chapter 7

1. They are called cyanoacrylates

2. alcohol, water, and weak alkaline (bases) substances.

3. lower or weaker

4. weave, thickness

5. Safety glasses, mist masks, and proper ventilation

6. oligomer

7. Thickness of gel layer, length of cure, bulb condition, and type of oligomer.

8. a. most likely

9. Any trauma to the nail plate can lead to separation (i.e., overfiling, heavy abrasives and drills, overpriming and wearing enhancements that are too long).

10. No one type of nail enhancement product is better for the nail plate than another!

Chapter 8

1. Both say that everything can be dangerous if you overexpose yourself to that substance.

2.
   - Potentially hazardous ingredients found in each product
   - Proper storage and fire prevention
   - Ways to prevent hazardous chemicals from entering your body
   - The short- and long-term health effects of overexposure
   - Early warning signs of product overexposure
   - Emergency first aid advice
   - Emergency phone numbers
   - Safe handling techniques

3. a. *Inhalation* of vapors, mists and dusts.

   b. *Absorption* through the skin or broken tissue.

   c. Accidental or unintentional *ingestion.*

4. Keep caps on containers and empty trash often.

5. Vapors are hundreds of times smaller than dust particles.

6. Overexposure can cause headaches, nausea, angry or frustrated feelings, nosebleeds, coughs, dizziness, tingling fingers and toes, dry or scratchy nose and throat, puffy red and irritated skin, itching, and many other symptoms.

7. exposure, safe levels.

8. 0%—all substances can be toxic.

9. No, nature is a dangerous place filled with potentially harmful substances. Many natural substances are more hazardous than their synthetic counterparts.

10. Put on your safety glasses.

Chapter 9

1. Skin diseases.

2. Corrosives can cause permanent damage; irritations will usually disappear when overexposure discontinues.

3. Irritants cannot cause lifetime allergic reactions and sensitizers do.

4. Water and methacrylic acid primer.

5. Exaggerated or extreme sensitivity to a substance that lasts for life.

6. Vinyl, natural latex, polyethylene, polyurethane, and nitrile could also answer PVA and neoprene.

7. weak

8. sensitizer, allergen

9. Avoid prolonged and repeated contact or overexposure to the skin.

Chapter 10

1. Olfactory fatigue

2. breathing zone

3. dappen dish

4. It must clean your breathing zone.

5. High concentrations of ozone may cause eye, throat, and lung irritation.

6. Vapor molecules are hundreds of times smaller than dust particles. They whiz right through a HEPA filter.

7. It is a type of ventilation system that captures vapors, mists, and dust at the source and expels them from your breathing zone.

8. 50-100

9. 15 feet

10. Activated charcoal

Index

G

Gel lights, 99-100
Gels, 47, 78, 97-98, 103-104
Gloves, 134-136. *See also* Safety
Glues, 37, 93-94
Growth of nail plate. *See* Nail plate

H

Half-moon (lunula), 5
Handling chemicals, 113. *See also* Safety
Hardness, 20
Health effects from overexposure, 112
Heat energy, 51
Heat-curing, 52
HEPA filters, 146
High Efficiency Particle Filters. *See* HEPA filters
Homopolymer, 72
Hyponychium, 8

I

Infections, 102, 132, 135-136
Infrared light. See Heat energy
Ingestion (eating) potentially hazardous chemicals, 111, 116-117.
    See also Safety
Inhalation (breathing) potentially hazardous chemicals, 111. *See also* Safety
Inhibitors, 77-78
Initiator, 47, 51, 53, 70, 99
Interpenetrating Polymer Network. *See* IPNs
Ionizers, 147
IPNs, 50-51
Irritant contact dermatitis, 128

K

Keratin, 4, 15, 17, 21

L

Lateral nail fold, 3